Ten Follies: A Journey Around the World in Ten Forms of Madness

Ten Follies: A Journey Around the World in Ten Forms of Madness focuses on a critical question in the history of psychiatry: to what extent does psychopathology describe phenomena that exist before or beyond their description? Marco Innamorati probes the view that any description of a psychopathological phenomenon is, to a significant extent, the result of a construction by the subject describing it or a co-construction made by the clinician and the patient – a perspective also known as the "constructivist" approach.

Starting from the work of the philosopher and historian of science Ian Hacking, who proposed the concept of "transient mental illness", i.e., an "illness that appears at a given time, in a given place, and then disappears" (Hacking, 1998), Innamorati explores some forms of madness that seem to arise in a particular environment and specific historical circumstances, developing through a kind of epidemic and then disappearing almost definitively. The author evaluates strengths and weaknesses of the "constructivist" approach, by juxtaposing evolving hermeneutical questions to cultural factors. From hysteria to demonic possession, from the "mad travellers" to arctic shamanism, until the recent mushrooming of the hikikomori phenomenon,

Ten Follies is an unconventional "journey around the world in ten forms of madness" which takes the reader through astonishing stories of suffering and healing. Against the trend of mapping a single globalised discourse of "folly", this book embraces a kind of philosophical perspectivism ("ten follies") which echoes the contemporary cultural transformation of the many narratives of "madness".

Marco Innamorati is full professor of History and Philosophy of Scientific Concepts and Dynamic and Developmental Psychology at the University of Rome "Tor Vergata", Italy. He already published for Routledge *A Critical History of Psychotherapy*, Volume 1 and 2 (with Renato Foschi).

GLOBAL PERSPECTIVES ON THE HISTORY OF NATURAL PHILOSOPHY

Global Perspectives on the History of Natural Philosophy

Series Editors:
Yael Kedar (Tel Hai College, Israel), Cecilia Panti (University of Rome Tor Vergata, Italy) and Nicola Polloni

Fostering a new approach to the study of the history of natural philosophy this series aims to expand the discussion on natural philosophy cross-culturally and comparatively by focusing on the philosophical reasoning about nature developed particularly, but not exclusively, in three main cultural settings: Europe, the Middle East, and China. One of the main focal points of *Global Perspectives on the History of Natural Philosophy* is the interplay between philosophical and scientific concepts, stances, and problems arising from the premodern consideration of nature, broadly considered. Accordingly, the series provides a cutting-edge framework in which natural philosophy can be considered from new philosophically meaningful angles. Acknowledging the historical interweaving of philosophy and science of nature, the series publishes monographs and edited volumes dealing with the history of natural philosophy from three methodological perspectives: philosophical analysis, historical reconstruction, and comparative studies. Submitted manuscripts may either examine authors and issues from a specific philosophical tradition or engage comparatively with patterns and problems shared by different cultural settings.

Dante's Visions
Crossing Sights on Natural Philosophy, Theory of Vision, and Medicine in the Divine Comedy and Beyond
Edited by Cecilia Panti and Marco Piccolino

Mathematics and Philosophy at the Turn of the First Millennium
Abbo of Fleury on *Calculus*
Clelia V. Crialesi

Aristotle and New Spain
Virginia Aspe Armella

Ten Follies: A Journey Around the World in Ten Forms of Madness
Marco Innamorati

Ten Follies: A Journey Around the World in Ten Forms of Madness

Marco Innamorati

Routledge
Taylor & Francis Group
LONDON AND NEW YORK

First published in English 2025
by Routledge
4 Park Square, Milton Park, Abingdon, Oxon OX14 4RN

and by Routledge
605 Third Avenue, New York, NY 10158

Routledge is an imprint of the Taylor & Francis Group, an informa business

Translated by Tommaso Priviero

Published in Italian by Edizioni Unicopli 2021

British Library Cataloguing-in-Publication Data
A catalogue record for this book is available from the British Library

ISBN: 978-1-032-77101-4 (hbk)
ISBN: 978-1-032-77102-1 (pbk)
ISBN: 978-1-003-48124-9 (ebk)

DOI: 10.4324/9781003481249

Typeset in Sabon
by KnowledgeWorks Global Ltd.

Contents

Acknowledgement

The translation of the book was possible thanks to the contribution of the Department of History, Humanities and Society of the University of Rome Tor Vergata and the Centro Studi Europa e Umanesimo – Radici d'Occidente.

Introduction

0.1 Basic Principles

What is mental illness? We often hear the answer that it is the manifestation of an abnormality of the brain. This is correct in the sense that our mind is certainly an expression of brain activity. According to some, it can even be *identified* with such activity. However, the brain is not limited to the transmission of chemical and electrical impulses within the physiological environment constituted by the body: the human being also interacts with the external environment, which is of fundamental importance for the formation of the personality and its possible abnormalities.

Our personality is partly based on *temperament*, i.e. innate tendencies,[1] and partly on *experience*, i.e. the relationships we have with other people.[2] Without "Thou", there is no "I", as the philosopher Martin Buber wrote,[3] meaning that without contact with others, we simply would not exist as human beings. The ability itself to use language is only acquired because a subject is exposed to words in the nurturing environment.

Similarly, various animals also require parental care at the beginning of their existence and need a social context to survive. However, these relational aspects are essentially linked to instinct, i.e. *species-specific* (characteristic of the species) behaviours that are standardised.[4] In general, they evolve in a limited way and do not give rise to a fully formed *culture*, although it has been ascertained that, for example, adaptation to the city environment can lead some bird species to change their "songs".[5] It will therefore be no more difficult for a monkey that has lived in a German zoo to communicate with another monkey of the same species from a British zoo than with a similar monkey raised elsewhere in Germany. In fact, even monkeys raised in complete isolation are capable of producing the standard communicative signals of their own species, although the mode and correct timing of emission are the result of learning.[6] It has also been observed that individuals can occasionally *invent* specific communicative signals.[7]

Human cultural diversities are not limited to communicative signals but involve modes of interaction, customs, symbols, and activities with specific

DOI: 10.4324/9781003481249-1

functions. Even mental health and mental illness show similarities and differences in specific cultural contexts.

So-called descriptive psychopathology, as a discipline aimed at classifying mental disorders in a common, at least partly standardised language, was born during the 19th century[8] and has, according to many authors, retained a relative, although in some ways surprising, stability over the last century and a half.[9] If, however, the different forms of disorders (of thought, perception, memory, etc.) have been classified by Euro-Western psychiatrists in a fairly similar manner over time, very different have been the theoretical perspectives adopted to explain the origin of the disorders themselves, their immediate causes, and the significance and importance of the symptoms that characterise them.

The various attempts to offer an *objective* description of psychopathology have always been contested. On the one hand, since 19th century Franco-German psychiatry, the hope of identifying a correspondence between brain lesions and diseases of the mind has only found partial and limited confirmation. On the other hand, the attempt to establish a *phenomenology* of mental illness, i.e. an objective reconstruction of the inner experience of the mentally ill, from Jaspers[10] onwards clashes with the already enormous difficulty of a *phenomenological* understanding of humanity as such. Fascinating as Husserl's and Heidegger's attempts in this regard may have been, their psychological application has generally been limited, if not received with coldness and detachment.[11] Moreover, phenomenological psychiatry has found it extremely difficult to find mentally ill persons capable of rendering their experience of illness with sufficient breadth, in a way that can be used by the clinician, especially in the context of the most severe pathologies.[12]

Finally, the claim to offer an a-theoretical description of mental illness, that is, a description independent of reference theories, remains strongly contested. We will return to this point several times in the course of this book. For now, we will simply point out that philosophers of science have long since made it clear that it is not possible to observe pure facts without presuppositions. Facts are always theory-laden[13] and the claim of pure observation has ironically been called "immaculate perception" by Nietzsche.[14]

Today, the idea that simply "diseases of the mind are diseases of the brain"[15] seems to have been definitively abandoned. Far from being abandoned, instead, seems to be the perspective according to which the authentic description of any psychopathological symptom is reducible to the "interaction between a tenuous biological *signal* (originating in an affected brain site) and the layers of psychosocial codes (noise) partaking in the process of symptom formation".[16] However, since it can be observed that only in the presence of *certain layers of the social codes* are certain symptoms formed, this perspective must necessarily change. Thus, the internal and external environment must, as mentioned above, be given equal importance in contributing to human conduct. This perspective undermines the debate on the *embodiment* of mental illness, i.e. the discussion of whether suffering is borne by the mind or the body, which has not only concerned organicists such as Griesinger and his successors, but also psychoanalysis since Freud and phenomenology.[17] In fact, individuals should necessarily be considered in the *field* that is constituted by their interpersonal interactions.[18]

Starting from this, this book explores a number of mental illnesses which seem to depend on specific historical, geographical and social conditions. It evaluates the hypothesis that what is considered a mental illness in one time and place may not be considered such elsewhere, in another era. The word *madness* will be understood here in the broad sense, as any condition that causes psychological suffering to the person being diagnosed, categorised or sometimes stigmatised. The application of a label, in fact, can sometimes be more damaging than the condition itself which the label describes.

This book addresses a key epistemological question: to what extent does psychopathology describe phenomena that exist *prior to* their description and *independently* of it? And to what extent is the opposite point of view acceptable? Namely, that every description of a psychopathological phenomenon is the result of the *construction* by the person describing it, or the *co-construction* operated by the clinician and the patient? In other words, the question arises to what extent is a *realist* approach possible (whereby it would be possible in principle to describe objectively what is observed) or is a *constructivist* approach appropriate (whereby all knowledge would in fact be the result of construction by a theorist).

Between these two poles, other perspectives are possible. For example, the metaphor of the "hermeneutic circle"[19] should be mentioned, which conceives knowledge as ultimately bound to a self-foundation, whereby knowledge is provisional, if not illusory. Another perspective is the metaphor of science as a building erected on piles,[20] whereby, although provisional and precarious, theoretical edifices become stabilised by experience, while proceeding by trial and error.

A direct inspiration for this book is the work of the philosopher and historian of science Ian Hacking, who proposed the concept of "transient mental illness", i.e. "an illness that appears at a given time, in a given place, and then disappears".[21] Hacking, who tends decidedly towards constructivism, in fact noted that some forms of madness seem to arise in a particular environment and under particular historical circumstances, experience a kind of epidemic and then disappear almost permanently.

In order to be able to speak of a mental illness, it is necessary to be able to identify people who *suffer* from it; people who *describe* their suffering; *conditions* that induce that suffering and *motives* that drive a person to evade reality in that particular way. We will provisionally take suffering for granted. It is less obvious that description is not only necessary for one to know about it but has a decisive influence on suffering people. Hacking speaks in this regard of a *looping effect*. On the one hand, if people are labelled in a certain way, they will already tend to behave in accordance with that label, especially if the labeller is perceived as an authority (scientific, religious etc.). On the other hand, the *stigma* will contribute to isolating people, who may in turn isolate themselves in order not to meet the condemning and scorning looks of others.

The cultural and environmental conditions that determine the emergence of a mental illness are different in different contexts and also contribute indirectly to its expression, influencing both the description by specialists and the reasons for the *choice* of that mental illness. The idea of "choosing" a mental illness might sound paradoxical to the non-specialist reader. In fact, the expression was coined by Freud[22] to identify an issue that appeared extremely problematic to him: what leads a person to present a certain symptom rather than another? Since it is not a conscious choice, the assumption of psychoanalytic theory was that it is unconscious motive that lead to it.

Hacking has devoted two monographs to two instances of "transient mental illness": mad travellers and multiple personality. Both will be illustrated in chapters in this book. Hacking's perspective, however, has important precedents, and certainly not only from a constructivist point of view. The birth of depth psychology is linked to the ideas of the *meaning* of symptoms and the *secondary gain* of illness. Sigmund Freud posited that the apparent strangeness of the mentally ill person is linked to the *conflict* that occurs within them between opposing tendencies: for example, the impulse to satisfy certain desires and the fear of the possible consequences of those actions. The conflict can lead a person to perform acts that constitute a *compromise* between the different tendencies. Freud also believed that the reason why it is difficult to recover from a mental illness is that, although the sufferer loses his or her ability to live fully, they *can* also receive a paradoxical compensation from it (the pursuit of which is completely unconscious). It should be recalled at this point that, as much as Hacking tends towards perspectivism, Freud was a firm believer in scientific realism, and he considered the realist perspective to be the only postulate necessary to accept psychoanalysis.[23] This has not prevented psychoanalysis from also developing hermeneutic foundation hypotheses[24] or "third ways" between science and hermeneutics.[25]

For some, madness may be the alternative to awareness of a reality that one cannot accept because it appears too unpleasant or even terrifying. A child's mental illness may force a parental couple otherwise close to splitting up to unity and solidarity, and so the child may be somewhat compensated for his or her impairment by the fact that the parents do not separate. A person's mental illness may be so severe as to constitute grounds for a disability pension; it is not uncommon for such a pension to constitute the sole source of family income – what then will be the motivation of this person to improve? Systemic psychotherapists believe that cases in which the family system can obtain a kind of equilibrium from the suffering of one of its members are by no means uncommon, so they define the mentally ill person as the *identified patient* (i.e. a family member who is used as an expression or a kind of scapegoat for the family's internal conflicts). It is thus understood that it is the family as a whole that actually chooses one of its members as a sort of grounding of all the tensions and problems that actually affect family relationships.[26]

Carl Gustav Jung as well had already realised that the different ways of describing mental illnesses are anything but objective: they depend on the personality of the psychologists, or rather on their *psychological type* (just as the most appropriate therapy would also depend on the psychological type).[27]

Moreover, long before Hacking expounded his ideas, the psychologist and philosopher Erich Fromm had already theorised the concept of "social character", meaning that certain personality characteristics tend to be shared by the majority of a population as history evolves.[28] Fromm was convinced, on the one hand, that social character changes significantly over time. On the other hand, it is not always adaptive to the given conditions of existence in a particular era. When social character clashes with the possibility of adaptation to the context, the conditions for revolutionary upheaval are created, according to Fromm. These are exceptions, however, and it is more likely, instead, that not sharing the social character is a source of discomfort for the individual: this could, in fact, be the reason why the conditions for transient mental illness are created.

Fromm constituted one of the most distinguished exponents of the Neo-Freudian movement, whose main characteristic was the attempt to relativise Freud's thought as a description of the psychology (and psychopathology) of a specific environment: the Victorian-minded West. In other words, Fromm and his colleagues, such as Harry Stack Sullivan, Karen Horney, and Clara Thompson, represented the psychological expression of the attempt already set up by anthropologists to move away from ethnocentrism, from the mentality according to which there would exist an objective point of view, that of the contemporary Western white man, in the face of which (any) other perspectives constitute deviations. Michel Foucault's controversial but important contribution,[29] which clearly informs Hacking, finally showed how madness can be made into a history, showing not only how society's attitude towards the insane has changed over time, but also how the forms of madness have changed. Histories of psychopathological symptoms have then been proposed, more recently, more or less systematically and for more or less extended periods, by other authors.[30]

In short, it has long been known that mental illness is not a random, psycho-physiological event with manifestations unrelated to the context. Instead, it is conditioned by where and when a person is born and how their peers interact with them or influence their lives. Just as it is known that the description of mental illness is not objective and influences those who suffer from it.

While the possibility of the existence of "transient mental illnesses" is worthy of attention, the phenomenon of mental illnesses that seem to be linked to a kind of *genius loci* is at least as significant: they were born in a certain area of the planet and have remained confined to that area, sometimes without there being any reason to think that the number of cases has increased or decreased significantly over time. Some of these mental illnesses represent isolated cases of cultures with precise boundaries, nevertheless constituting a locally known component of those cultures: this is the case of *Arctic hysteria*, an occupational disease of the shamans of the Far North. Others are characteristic of a very wide, but nevertheless defined area; *amok* is widespread in several areas of the Far East.

Between the mid-19th and early 20th century, a specific discipline was born that studied this kind of disorders, namely, *ethnopsychiatry*. Two different impulses initiated its formation process. In the United States, it was mainly a psychiatric prejudice. When, between 1839 and 1844, a wave of "new" migrants (predominantly Irish and German) poured into the country, the "old" inhabitants, especially those of British origin, tended to view them as "inferior". Mental health specialists speculated on the possibility that they were prone to different and arguably more difficult to treat psychopathologies. In the European context, however, it was the phenomenon of colonisation that started the process: when the colonial powers began to build institutions for the recovery of the mentally ill in the occupied countries, specialists began to observe the existence of previously unknown syndromes.[31]

Ethnopsychiatry has traditionally dealt with forms of pathology linked to "other" cultures, with the risk of "other" implicitly meaning "less developed". Only recently there has been a change in this trend, which led to the recognition that all forms of psychopathology should be defined as "culturally bound", including those that are, so to speak, classical and Western based.[32] In fact, anthropologists have long been fighting this risk, warning us that singularity and diversity belong to our own culture just as much as to others.

Conversely, there are rituals that serve the same function in different cultures, even though they are expressed in apparently very distant ways. For instance, Daniel Miller found unsuspected similarities in shopping and in rites of sacrifice and devotion present in less secularised contexts than in the contemporary West.[33] Similarly, different cultures express seemingly similar beliefs, but these may have quite different applications in their respective contexts. For example, "it means nothing that a magic practice of an African tribe has analogies with one in use in the Italian Renaissance, because the meaning, the efficacy of that practice *is not and cannot be*, by definition, that of Renaissance magic".[34]

Ethnopsychiatry and cultural anthropology also began, during the 20th century, to take an interest in forms of treatment specific to cultures other than the West. Taking his cue from these studies, Jerome Frank argued that there are more similarities between modern psychotherapy and more allegedly "primitive" forms of therapy than it seems on the surface.[35] Ellenberger explicitly asserted that the most archaic roots of Freud's, Jung's, and Adler's ideas derive precisely from that world of shamans and healers to which historians of psychotherapy had originally looked only with distracted curiosity.[36]

Finally, it should be noted that some forms of mental suffering appear to be originally linked to a particular culture, but subsequently spread elsewhere, where specific conditions for their spread are created. An example of this type is the *hikikomori*, which originated in Japan not a long time ago, but in recent years has also reached the West. That of the *hikikomori* is a very particular case because, as we shall see, the term itself seems to indicate mental conditions that in different cultural contexts take on forms with common elements, but discordant characteristics.

A common problem in the classification as well as in the diagnosis of mental illnesses is their *authenticity*. This can sometimes be a false problem because, as mentioned above, the description of the pathology is influenced both by the *person* suffering from it, the *specialist* observing it, and the *society* in which both live. With the case of *demonic possession*, for example, in the eyes of a lay scientist, the idea that a person can be penetrated and controlled by an evil spiritual entity may be completely meaningless. However, it cannot be doubted that in many historical contexts and even in many environments contemporary to us, possession has been considered a real phenomenon, to be treated as such. From this point of view, one should not forget the contributions of Ernesto De Martino, when he studied magic[37]and tarantism[38] in southern Italy as an anthropologist. The question is not whether a witch can really hover in the air by anointing herself with grease, nor whether a spider bite can be cured by dancing the tarantella. Rather, the question is what effects on popular life the belief that these were authentic facts entailed. Such effects are, indeed, real. As Ludwig Wittgenstein provocatively wrote, there is no reason to think that religious beliefs should not "make part of that inherited heritage on the basis of which I distinguish between true and false".[39]

The case of possession illustrates another characteristic of some forms of psychological suffering: the possibility of having different manifestations in different contexts. As will be seen in the relevant chapter, the relationship with a demon may be suffered, sought after, or experienced in a more or less tranquil coexistence, depending on the case. Another interesting aspect is related to possession: the same person may a priori consider the authenticity of the same phenomenon differently in different contexts. A Catholic priest might consider the efficacy of a rite performed by an exorcist to be proof that a demon has been cast out, but the same result obtained by a shaman would instead seem to him to be the fruit of popular credulity.

Probably some forms of "transient mental illness" in the sense indicated by Hacking are the result of a specific spatial and temporal condition but reflect a category of mental suffering with at least partly similar characteristics that may exist before and after the specific local epidemic. *Conversion hysteria* can probably be considered a transient mental illness in Hacking's sense, whereas hysteria *tout court* does not. It should be noted that so-called Arctic hysteria has nothing to do with either "Western" hysteria in general or conversion hysteria in particular: a similarity that only early observers thought they saw, hence the hasty translation of the term *pibloktok*.

If some mental illnesses can be classified as fictitious, in the sense that some people can simulate suffering from them, it is also possible that it is the specialists devoted to their description who simulate their existence. *Sluggish schizophrenia* is a specific case of this kind. The first generation of Soviet psychiatrists diagnosed it to dissidents in the USSR to please the regime, but of its reality as a nosographic entity few of their pupils of later generations ever doubted, until the fall of the so-called Iron Curtain.

In short, there are many different faces and masks of madness or, more generally, of psychic distress, so much so that their definition is very complicated.

0.2 Normal and Exceptional

In the *Confessions*, Augustine wrote the following about the meaning of the word "time": "Provided that no one asks me, I know".[40] Probably something similar could happen to those who attempt to unambiguously define the word "madness". The apparently easiest way would be to define it from its opposite: madness is a condition other than mental normality. Even the idea of "normality", however, has an ambiguous meaning. The word "normal" is derived from "norm", a legal term. Then "norm" is something that is established; it is a convention that regulates relations between people and divides what is legitimate from what is not. When it is applied to mental health, the idea of normality thus implicitly refers to an empirical metrics: there must be parameters on the basis of which it can be decided whether a specific behaviour, a mental characteristic, an existential conduct or, more generally, the personality of a human being falls within the canons established as "normality". Like jurisprudence, however, these canons are by no means eternal and fixed.

Moreover, the reference point of "normality" is itself interpretable in different ways. First of all, there is the issue of a person's self-perception in relation to the perception that others have of that person. Subjectively, a person may consider as normal a condition that he or she has lost, something that others would consider out of the norm. For example, an accident might cause a racing pilot to lose the absolute tranquillity that characterised them driving at 300 km/h. In the eyes of such a driver, returning to driving with the previous coolness would mean returning to normality, while in the eyes of other human beings, there would be nothing normal about the same condition. One could, of course, argue that these are exceptional cases, but even if one turns to a more broadly shared conception of normality, one is still far from an unambiguous view.

One could then use as synonyms for normality the ideal condition, the average, or the majority. The first option may not appear obvious and to introduce it better a comparison between the mental and medical spheres is appropriate. When one undergoes a check-up, a large number of examinations can be performed, analysing the body fluids and investigating the appearance and functionality of the various organs. Normality is defined in that context as the condition in which every element investigated describes the body as fully functional. But is it so obvious that *all* results correspond to normality? Apparently not. It is worth recalling a paradox that each of us implicitly accepts without thinking too much about it: frequently we hear, for example, "it is normal that at a certain age..." In fact, this means that it is normal for there to be abnormality.

Similarly, psychic normality would consist of a state in which a person knows how to adapt to whatever situation they are faced with in the course of their existence, has satisfying and profound interpersonal relationships, is devoid of conflicts and inhibitions, and always maintains perfect control of their aggression. Lucio Dalla, a famous Italian songwriter, used to wittily sing "*Ma la cosa veramente eccezionale, credi, — è essere normale!*" ("The really exceptional thing, believe me, is to be normal!"). In this perspective, he was probably right. If we think of a "perfect" normality, few human beings fall within it. It is therefore a limiting concept, not easy to apply, and of relative usefulness.

We can then think of normality as referring rather to the average condition of the population. Certain aspects of a person's psychology are in principle measurable (with a pinch of salt). For example, if one defines intelligence in terms of performance, normal intelligence is that which corresponds to average performance in intelligence tests. Conventionally, a value of 100 would then correspond to normality, while "out of the norm" in a positive or negative sense would be values far above or far below 100. However, very few features of the human mind are equally measurable; not to mention that the numerical value can vary significantly depending on the performance being measured. Moreover, when considering mental health, we usually refer to phenomena in terms of presence/absence.

Normal could be accordingly defined, then, as an attitude, a trait, a behaviour that is characteristic of most people or at least of a significant part of the population. However, we are forced to admit that on certain historical occasions what was common to the majority of a population is considered abnormal today, or at least not considered normal.

For instance, the Germans' adherence to Nazism in the 1930s is now counted among the examples of a people's collective transient madness. The belief that slavery was a humanly acceptable condition was prevalent for a long time in Western civilisation, as much as the female subjection to men in patriarchal societies. However, if the benchmark is the present, it is evident that what seems normal to us today may appear abnormal tomorrow to other peoples or in other cultural contexts. Paradoxically, psychological suffering may be normal on the basis of the sharing principle: if not the majority of human beings, a very significant proportion of them have suffered from episodes of depression during their lives. We should therefore consider depression as normal, which seems counterintuitive.

A somewhat eccentric view, but one that cannot be excluded a priori in the context of the present discussion, is what has been called the "psychedelic" concept of normality[41]. The well-known and much-discussed psychiatrist Ronald Laing argued that the society in which we live is so alienating, that most people adapt to it because their minds are limited, and the only true normal people would be the insane.[42]

At any rate, using the majority as a reference presents a serious problem: *minority characteristics risk being classified as abnormal precisely because they are not shared by common sense.* When slavery of African-Americans was considered a natural condition, the fact that some slaves escaped from the cotton plantations of the U.S. South aspiring to freedom was considered insane. The runaway slave suffered from *drapetomania.*[43] But, of course, the most dramatic example in this area is homosexuality. Homosexual relationships were considered by all means normal in Ancient Greece. The most important Greek texts on eros, Plato's *Symposium* and Plutarch's *Dialogue On Love*, discuss whether or not a man's love for a woman is as noble as that for another man, offering, at least the former, an entirely negative answer. Nevertheless, from the moment homosexuality was described as a form of *perversion* (in the 19th century), until most of the last century, homosexual love in the West was discouraged, despised, socially sanctioned, or even criminally punished by the majority. Even today there are psychiatrists and psychologists (thankfully a minority) who believe it is possible and appropriate to "cure" homosexuality.

0.3 Madness and Psychological Distress

"All happy families are alike, every unhappy family is unhappy in its own way". So goes one of the most famous opening lines in the history of literature, that of Tolstoy's *Anna Karenina.* Different forms of family "unhappiness" can generally be traced back to different forms of psychological distress of their members. It would seem already established at this point that mental suffering has different modes of expression or, in the language we have used, different faces and masks. It would be appropriate now to point out that it also has different levels of *severity*, that is, it can be more or less disabling.

Until the time when psychiatry aspired to specifically characterise the various forms of mental illness, there was a tendency to make a clear distinction between *clinical* and *non-clinical* conditions. There existed, even in the eyes of technicians, on the one hand, the normal person and on the other the insane person, who deserved visible treatment or at least distinction from the rest of society, which was not always negative. In some cultures, madness was able to attribute a kind of privilege to those affected by it. In the Greek language, the terms denoting madness (*mania*) and the ability to predict the future (*mantiké*) have the same etymological root,[44] testifying to the fact that it was the person considered insane who assumed the role of oracle/sibyl. Similarly, shamans were often chosen for mental characteristics that would have caused them isolation elsewhere.

On the contrary, the attempt to classify mental illnesses developed in parallel with the increasingly precise conviction, first, of the existence of forms of distress milder than proper madness (the so-called "neuroses"), but nevertheless deserving of therapy; then, of a real continuity between normal and pathological. The latter opinion was shared by the fathers of contemporary psychotherapy: Janet, Freud, Adler, and Jung. We will not dwell on the reasons why perhaps today there is not complete unanimity on the question of whether the threshold between normality and pathology is only quantitative or rather qualitative.[45] As far as we now propose to illustrate, it will suffice for us to consider that such a threshold is in any case rather thin and that even normal people may occasionally exhibit conduct that momentarily distances them from normality. Of course, this "distance" from normality may be more or less substantial.

As is well known, Freud considered *parapraxes* to be symptoms and he spoke of them as *micro-neurotic phenomena*.[46] From the psychoanalytic point of view, if one hears a fellow say: "Now that we live close together, we can meet more seldom", instead of, as he would consciously like to say, "more often", one ascribes to this "involuntary mistake" a real intention in accordance with what in fact escaped from the person's mouth. One may or may not agree with Freud,[47] but certainly the Freudian slip is a departure from the norm. One does not have to be a psychoanalyst to realise that if a person does not come to an appointment with us and justifies themselves by saying that they *forgot*, that missed act tells us a lot about the consideration in which that person holds us.

The same "normal" person might, once in a lifetime, be involved in a fight and hit someone else hard. He or she might later say something like: "I don't know what happened to me: I wasn't really myself!" In this case, this person is using what in Perry's DMRS scale (Defence Mechanisms Rating Scale) is classified as dissociation: "a temporary alteration of the integrative functions of consciousness or identity".[48] This person would thus perceive the distance between the conduct they expect of themselves and the conduct they occasionally engage in. They would know that they had stepped outside the norm.

In any case, a threshold of normality seems to exist, and some seem to have crossed it permanently if it is said of them that *they suffer from a mental illness* (supposedly, a minority) and others not.

The criteria by which mental illness (and specifically insanity) is qualified as such are usually linked to two orders of factors: on the one hand, the symptoms, and on the other hand, the difficulties that the symptoms cause oneself or others. However, in some cases, the symptoms are considered as such by both the person presenting them and the observer; in other cases, they are not. The schizophrenic, who recounts their hallucinations, is usually made uncomfortable by them and hopes it will be possible to get rid of them. The neurotic, who cannot experience their sexuality because they feel anxiety every time they can have intercourse, seeks help so that the anxiety will leave them. Conversely, the obsessive personality, who controls every detail of their existence, may be unbearable to others but considers their own behaviour entirely logical. The antisocial personality, who divides the world into victims and executioners, feels no sense of guilt in performing acts of extreme violence: why, they think, should they become a victim?

When symptoms are considered such by both the subject and the observer, they are called *ego-dystonic*: thoughts and behaviours that are conflicting or dissonant with the needs and goals of the "ego". When the person presenting them does not dismiss their symptoms, they are called *ego-syntonic*: thoughts and behaviours are perceived as in harmony with the needs and goals of the "ego". The problem then, as already mentioned, would be to establish to what extent one has the right to consider the symptoms and to what extent one has the right to treat them, and how. This point, however, will be explored further in the conclusions.

For now, let us begin our journey, which will illustrate on the one hand the conditions that favoured the emergence of a mental illness or its identification; on the other hand, those that determined its spread, decline, modification, or the reasons why it is no longer diagnosed as such. We will also discuss whether and when a mental illness was fabricated or even invented by those who described it. Each chapter will be devoted to a specific form of mental distress, which will be introduced by a clinical history.

Notes

1 Rothbart et al., "Temperament and Personality".
2 Sroufe at al., "Conceptualizing the Role of Early Experience"; Kernberg and Caligor, "A Psychoanalytic Theory of Personality Disorders".
3 Buber, *Das dialogische Prinzip*.
4 Tinbergen, *The Study of Instinct*.
5 Luther and Derryberry, "Birdsongs Keep Pace with City Life".
6 Call and Tomasello, *The Gestural Communication of Apes and Monkeys*.
7 Goodall, *The Chimpanzees of Gombe*.
8 Goldstein, *Console and Classify*.
9 Berrios, *History of the Mental Symptoms*.
10 Jaspers, *General Psychopathology*.
11 Husserl, *Ideas Pertaining to a Pure Phenomenology*; Heidegger, *Sein und Zeit*.
12 Blankenburg, *Der Verlust der natürlichen Selbstverständlichkeit*.
13 Hanson, *Patterns of Discovery*.
14 Nietzsche, *Also sprach Zarathustra*.
15 Griesinger, *Mental Mathology and Therapy*, 9.
16 Berrios, *History of the Mental Symptoms*, 1.
17 Innamorati, *Freud*; Zaner, *The Problem of Embodiment*; Straus, *Phenomenological Psychology*.
18 Lewin, *A Dynamic Theory of Personality*.
19 Gadamer, *Wahrheit und Methode*.

20 Popper, *Logic of Scientific Discovery.*
21 Hacking, *Mad Travellers*, 11.
22 Freud, *Heredity*; *Further Remarks.*
23 Freud, *The Question.*
24 Foschi and Innamorati, *A Critical History of Psychotherapy.*
25 Strenger, *Between Hermeneutics and Science.*
26 Bertrando and Toffanetti, *Storia della terapia familiare.*
27 Jung, *Psychological Types*; see Innamorati, *Jung.*
28 Fromm, *The Fear of Freedom.*
29 Foucault, *History of Madness.*
30 See, e.g., Berrios, *History of the Mental Symptoms*; Porter, *Madness. A Brief History*; Pietikäinen, *Madness*; Scull, *Madness in Civilisation.*
31 Wittkower and Prince, "A Review of Transcultural Psychiatry".
32 APA, *DSM-5.*
33 Miller, *A Theory of Shopping.*
34 Galimberti, "Introduzione", xi.
35 Frank, *Persuasion and Healing.*
36 Ellenberger, *The Discovery of the Unconscious.*
37 De Martino, *Sud e magia.*
38 De Martino, *La terra del rimorso.*
39 Wittgenstein, *On Certainty*, 29.
40 Augustine of Hippo, *Confessions*, xi, 14, 17; p. 242.
41 Scharfetter, *General Psychopathology.*
42 Laing, *The Divided Self.*
43 Cartwright, "Report on the Diseases and Physical Peculiarities of the Negro Race".
44 Liddell and Scott, *A Greek-English Lexicon.*
45 See a discussion of this issue in Lenzenweger and Clarkin (Eds.), *Major Theories of Personality Disorder.*
46 Freud, *The Psychopathology of Everyday Life.*
47 See, e.g., Timpanaro, *Il lapsus freudiano.*
48 Perry, *Defense Mechanism Rating Scales*; Di Giuseppe and Perry, "The Hierarchy of Defence Mechanisms".

1 Conversion Hysteria

1.1 The Story of Bertha, Alias Anna O.

One summer evening in 1882, Bertha Pappenheim, an upper-middle-class woman in Vienna, suffered terribly from the heat but cannot drink a drop of water. The very idea of raising a glass to her mouth disgusts her and she cannot explain why. The only way to escape her thirst is to eat fresh fruit, but it is an admittedly impractical method. This symptom has been haunting her for some time and in the summer heat it has become unbearable. In the evenings, she falls into a state of self-induced hypnosis, during which she is able to recall events apparently forgotten during her waking state and talk about them with her neurologist, Joseph Breuer, who visits her regularly. Thus, Bertha recalls that months earlier she had seen her lady-in-waiting offer water from her own glass to the little dog. For Bertha, that dog was an unclean beast. Due to her politeness and etiquette, Bertha had not at the time vented the anger and disgust she felt upon seeing the scene, but she can now unburden herself by recalling it. While recounting the episode, Bertha pounces on a glass of water and drinks greedily. She wakes up from hypnosis and continues drinking, apparently free of this symptom once and for all.

Hydrophobia was not the only symptom that Bertha presented when Breuer began to follow her. Ever since her father – whom she adored – had fallen seriously ill and died, she had begun to present an intricate symptomatologic picture, for which apparently no physical, medical reasons could be found. Contracture paresis, anaesthesia in various parts of the body, disturbances of vision and hearing, neuralgia, coughing, tremors, and even inability to express herself in her own language. Bertha is able to speak to her doctor in English, but if she wants to, she remains able to read Latin and speak French as before the illness. All these symptoms seem to be diagnosable as *hysterical* in Breuer's opinion. The neurologist, however, has a brilliant idea at this point: it may be that each symptom can be traced back to a specific event and that recalling that event brings with it the same liberating effect as the first recall! The credit for this insight, however, must be given as much to the doctor as to the patient. Here is what Breuer writes about it:

DOI: 10.4324/9781003481249-2

> These findings—that in the case of this patient the hysterical phenomena disappeared as soon as the event which had given rise to them was reproduced in her hypnosis-made it possible to arrive at a therapeutic technical procedure which left nothing to be desired in its logical consistency and systematic application. Each individual symptom in this complicated case was taken separately in hand; all the occasions on which it had appeared were described in reverse order, starting before the time when the patient became bed-ridden and going back to the event which had led to its first appearance. When this had been described the symptom was permanently removed.[1]

The technique works but turns out to be more difficult to implement than expected. Since the episode of the little dog drinking from the glass was only recalled in a hypnotic state, it becomes necessary for the patient to re-enter it every time she tries to evoke a new traumatic memory. Breuer discovers that intentionally hypnotising the girl presents no particular difficulty. It is enough for Bertha to experience a sensory impression that evokes the period to be remembered for her to sink into the hypnotic reminiscence. During the previous year, Bertha had mainly fed on oranges, and it is enough to present her with an orange to lead her hypnotically to recount episodes from 1881. A major difficulty, however, is that in order to be able to recall the first time a certain symptom appeared, Bertha needs to recall exactly in the right order, from the last to the first, all the occasions on which it occurred. Slowly, however, the process goes on and seems to work. Bertha, who seems to derive great relief from this, coins for her dialogues under hypnosis with Breuer two expressions that will make history: *chimney sweeping* and, above all, *talking cure*, which will in time become synonymous with *psychoanalysis*.

This story is told by Joseph Breuer to a young neurologist, Sigmund Freud, who at first does not attach too much importance to it. Freud, however, has the opportunity to meet the international star of neurology at the time, Jean-Martin Charcot, during a semester of lectures devoted to hysteria. Charcot does indeed use hypnosis on hysterics, but only for observational and not therapeutic purposes. Freud tells Charcot about Breuer's experience at this point, leaving the Frenchman completely indifferent. He does not lose heart, however, because he has intuited that Breuer's technique has important potential for therapeutic application. He begins hypnotising hysterical patients, being convinced of the traumatic origin of their disorder and of the possibility that the trauma has been "forgotten" (*repressed*, to use the term that would later be distinctively adopted by psychoanalysis) and that recalling it could allow the symptoms to be remitted. The attempts lead to partial successes and are recounted in a book signed by both Freud and Breuer, *Studies on Hysteria*. In this book, Breuer tells for the first time in a published text the story of his treatment of Bertha Pappenheim, whose name he covers with a pseudonym. Bertha becomes the patient zero of psychoanalysis, with the notorious alias of Anna O.

Breuer, however, ends his account hastily, stating that Bertha/Anna has been freed of all symptoms and that the cure therefore ended when it needed to end. In reality, 30 years after the publication of *Studies on Hysteria*, Freud came to a rather different conclusion. At the end of an umpteenth hypnosis session, the patient had tried to embrace an embarrassed Breuer. The latter had therefore decided to sever all contact with his patient and to leave immediately for a pleasure trip with his wife, a sort of second honeymoon.[2] From Freud's point of view, therefore, the story of Bertha and Josef became the first occasion on which a therapist was confronted with the problems induced by the phenomenon of *transference*, the special relationship established in therapy, which can result in falling in love with the therapist. Others have considered the same story as the first example of the damage caused by psychoanalysis.[3]

1.2 Hysteria in Continental Europe in the Late 19th and Early 20th Century

The history of hysteria is a peculiar one, because depending on the point of view, it can be considered extremely long or remarkably short. The history is long if one considers how long it has been described as a form of pathology with changing physical symptoms, the reality of which one always remains somewhat uncertain; a pathology generally diagnosed in female persons, so much so that it is often described in terms that seem to represent a kind of caricature of femininity. The story is short, instead, if one narrows it down to the period when there was a sort of epidemic of hysteria, with specific and spectacular symptoms, described in particular by Jean-Martin Charcot in Paris and Sigmund Freud in Vienna. According to most historians (not all of them), the epidemic mainly concerned continental Europe at the turn of the late 19th and early 20th century. Some people think that the hysterical disorder was always or almost always fictitious; others, that it disappeared during the last century; or that it simply changed its mode of manifestation.

The term "hysteria" has ancient roots. Its etymology refers to the word "uterus" and thus essentially characterised it as a female disease. Hysteria is defined as such by the school of Hippocrates, who first named it in this way, in the 5th century BC. However, a similar syndrome is described in Egyptian papyri dating back to 1900 BC.[4] Vague symptoms are attributed to hysterical illness: spasms, convulsions, and abnormal sensations of all kinds that come and go, simulating various different illnesses. One symptom that almost always occurs seems to be a sensation of suffocation or strangulation, which also comes and goes depending on the moment. The idea of Hippocrates is that the cause of this symptom (and of hysteria in general) is the property of the uterus to be able to move inside the body, reaching almost to the throat. As is well known, the Hippocratic doctrines, through the mediation of Galen, formed the basis of Western medicine for tens of centuries, and thus the conception of hysteria also remained essentially unchanged until the

Renaissance. Even when the belief that the uterus was mobile was discarded, however, the syndrome continued to be observed. Then the idea that the uterus was ascending into the oesophagus was replaced by the proposal that the choking sensation could be described as the presence of a reflux-phantasy of pre-digested food, hence the name "hysterical bolus".

Between the 17th and 18th century, hysteria began to be defined as a general disease of the nerves, between reality and simulation, a kind of female equivalent of hypochondria, which instead was characterised as typically male. Both hypochondria and hysteria were often classified among the afflictions caused by breathing unhealthy vapours.[5] Between the 18th and 19th century, further symptoms were attributed to hysteria: fainting, paralysis of different parts of the body, coughing, trance-like states, paraesthesia (loss of skin sensitivity); symptoms that were always temporary and tended to migrate from one part of the body to another.[6]

However, "classic" hysteria, which Freud defined as "conversion hysteria",[7] only became the subject of particular attention in the late 19th century, due to the remarkable increase in diagnoses, at least in France. According to the registers of the two main hospitals in Paris, Bicêtre, and Salpêtrière, the percentage of hysteria diagnoses among female in-patients rose from around 1% between 1841 and 1842 to more than 20% between 1882 and 1883.[8] In short, hysteria became a visible and significant phenomenon to the point that, a posteriori, in 1928, the Surrealists proposed celebrating the 50th anniversary of its *birth* in 1878. This date coincided with the creation of the photographic archive of the Salpêtrière, in which images of hysterical women under hypnosis began to be preserved. For prominent figures of the Surrealist movement such as Aragon and Breton,[9] hysteria had even become an art form.

To understand this phenomenon, one must take into account different historical events, although they can be linked to each other. The first event is the impetus, which came from France, of the disciplines that study mental illness: psychiatry and neurology. The first hero of French psychiatry was Philippe Pinel, who boasted of having "freed the insane from their chains", i.e. of having been the first to think that madness was not just a problem to be limited by imprisonment, but a state to be modified by therapy. The generation following Pinel, whose main exponent was Esquirol, began to classify the different forms of madness, trying to understand their origins and modulate their treatment. In French medicine, meanwhile, a principle was establishing itself, which, although it later proved to be only partially correct, provided fundamental momentum for the transformation of an empirical discipline into a true science. This was the so-called "Broussais principle" (coined by the philosopher Auguste Comte), which establishes that disease is not a condition qualitatively different from health: what changes is only a quantitative alteration in the activity of the body's organs. The success in applying this principle to various diseases was spectacular, particularly in the case of Claude Bernard (one of the fathers of modern medicine). The principle was then also applied to mental conditions, according to which the difference between insanity and normality must in turn be a quantitative difference and not a qualitative one. A certain amount of abnormality can reside in every person – an idea which will become one of the foundations of psychoanalysis. This, however, leads scholars to devote specific attention to a whole band of conditions that do not qualify as true "madness", but neither do they qualify as total "normality", namely, those that are indicated in general as "neurosis". They are still thought to be affections of the nerves, but less serious than "psychoses".

In this sense, hysteria went on to be given a privileged object of attention as a neurosis *par excellence*. As a matter of fact, hysteria progressively lost in the eyes of specialists the appearance of a rare disease in order to be diagnosed, as we have seen, in an ever-increasing number of people. It was believed that the symptoms must, to some extent, be traceable to the nervous system: where in the nervous system exactly; however, it did not seem easy to establish. In particular, certain symptoms go against all anatomical logic, now that the distribution of afferent and efferent nerves in the brain is beginning to seem quite clear. For example, a symptom characteristic of hysteria such as "glove" paralysis (affecting only one hand) contradicts the general principle that if one extremity is paralysed, the whole part of the body affected by the nerves reaching that extremity should be paralysed. If the hand is paralysed, the whole arm should be paralysed.

One person who particularly focused on hysteria was the aforementioned Jean-Marie Charcot, who possibly should be considered the true founder of scientific neurology,[10] but who owes his enormous popularity during his lifetime precisely to his studies on hysteria. His theory, in this regard, was that hysteria must be a disease with a hereditary predisposition. Since it only arises in adults, however, there must be a reason for its onset in the individual history of the sufferer. This reason can be identified in a *psychic trauma*, i.e. an episode that produces a strong impression on the potentially hysterical subject. According to Charcot, however, psychic trauma is not in itself the cause of hysteria, but only an *agent provocateur*. Just as the agent provocateur infiltrates a criminal or terrorist cell in order to induce it to action, so the psychic trauma would trigger the full-blown hysteria, which, however, is already there in power in the person's body, ready to be unleashed.

Thus, Charcot introduces a distinction between *grande hystérie* (grand hysteria), with a more florid symptomatology, characterised by strong "attacks", and *pétite hystérie* (small hysteria), which would be more limited. In his *Tuesday Lectures*, Charcot indicates a characteristic course of the attacks of grand hysteria: (1) a general stiffening of the sick person; (2) clonic convulsions, characterised by spectacular movements, which Charcot also referred to as "clownism"; (3) attitudes that seem to manifest intense passions (hatred, love, etc.); (4) a final delirium marked by tears, laughter or hiccups, which preludes a return to normality, with the exception of paraesthesia and paralysis.

According to Charcot, hysteria is also characterised by another symptom: a disposition to be easily *hypnotised*: only those suffering from hysteria could be hypnotised. Under hypnosis, they could also be induced to go through the various stages of the hysterical attack. Charcot begins to enrich his public lectures by hypnotising his patients, who "offer", so to speak, impressive demonstrations of their attacks in front of astonished spectators. In a short time, the fame of these unique shows spread and Charcot's lectures are attended by a large audience, including many important Parisian intellectuals. Some of Charcot's patients, like Blanche, become almost stars themselves. A real epidemic of hysteria begins.

There was no shortage of criticism of Charcot. Sceptics begin to suspect that the hysterical condition has advantages for the patients of the Salpêtrière, who belong to the poorer classes, and that some of them may have learnt to imitate the attacks of Blanche and her companions. Charcot responds to these criticisms, which historians now consider to be well-founded, as "very picturesque".

Hyppolite Bernheim rightly argues, in contrast to Charcot, that hypnotism is a characteristic that, although not universal, belongs to a much wider population than just hysterics. Under hypnosis, thanks to suggestion, anyone can be induced to manifest the symptoms of hysteria. Suggestions, however, can also be used for therapeutic purposes: patients suffering from mental illnesses can be induced under hypnosis to abandon their symptoms. Bernheim became the leading exponent of the Nancy School, which thus opposed the Salpêtrière School led by Charcot.[11] Bernheim's ideas, however well-founded, struggle to gain ground. After all, he is a provincial man criticising a Parisian luminary.

Freud also discovered Bernheim and spent a further period of formation abroad in Nancy. Compared to Bernheim and Charcot, however, Freud uses a third route to hypnosis. Whereas Charcot employed hypnosis for study purposes and Bernheim for suggestion, the founder of psychoanalysis uses it for catharsis. In fact, finally remembering forgotten traumas would allow, according to Freud a relief due to the dissolution of an accumulated and finally resolved tension.

Freud changes his approach from Charcot's on the aetiology of hysteria. In his view, psychic trauma is itself the cause. Those who suffer from hysteria suffer "mostly from reminiscences";[12] reminiscences which, however, are repressed in the person's *unconscious*. It should be remembered that Freud initially thought of a real trauma, such as violence suffered in childhood. Later, he attributed to the repressed fantasy the same traumatic value as an event that had actually occurred. What is thus repressed is, according to Freud, traceable to the sphere of sexuality. Indeed, it should be noted that while Charcot's patients are essentially from modest social backgrounds, the Viennese whom Freud treats belong to the bourgeois or upper middle class. In this sphere, the "civilised sexual morality" of the time obliges women to consider sexual life as something to be reserved for the sphere of marriage and, even in this context, functional to marital demands and the need to bear children. In that historical context, the idea of female sexual satisfaction is something to be considered improper and left to women of easy virtue. The higher social background of the Viennese patients presents a technical problem. If the indigent Parisians were willing to allow themselves to be hypnotised by Charcot with remarkable docility, this was less acceptable in the eyes of the bourgeois women under Freud's care.[13] Freud therefore abandoned hypnosis for what was to become the definitive psychoanalytic method: the use of the couch and the so-called "free association".

That sexual repression could be deeply problematic is, when Freud began his career, more than certain. Nor was Freud the first to realise that repressed sexuality can be the source of the most diverse psychopathological problems. On the one hand, there are numerous sexologists who were dealing with the issue in a systematic way, right up to the publication of Krafft-Ebing's monumental *Psychopathia sexualis*, which classified an impressive number of disorders that could be traced back to sexuality. On the other hand, it is Freud himself who admits that the problem had long been considered by doctors to be as well-known as unmentionable. A gynaecologist, in fact, had been able to send to him for treatment, a hysterical woman whose husband was impotent. The cure was, in his opinion, as obvious as it was difficult to prescribe: "*penis normalis dosim repetatur*" – "normal penis in repeated dosage".[14]

Freud, however, progressively draws general attention by attributing symptoms a specific meaning, of a symbolic nature. Symptoms, that is to say, can be regarded as *compromise formations* between two groups of mental forces, which remain outside consciousness: on the one hand, desires, on the other hand, a real *censorship*, the result of the morality of social conveniences that a person has absorbed through the education received. Thus, for example, a hysteric may experience gag reflexes at the thought of sexual intercourse, which on the one hand block its consummation, but on the other hand also evoke the possible effect of the act – the nausea of the pregnant person.[15] Or a hysteric struggling with the conflicting desire to hit his father with his fist finds himself with a paralysed arm.[16] Freud, therefore, begins to speak of "conversion hysteria", meaning that repressed sexuality is "converted" into symptoms. The treatment of hysteria becomes the workhorse of psychoanalysis.

At the end of the first decades of the 20th century, however, the epidemic of "conversion hysteria" with the manifestations described by Charcot and Freud, gradually subsided. It can certainly be stated that the spread of Freud's ideas throughout the West, especially between the 1910s and 1960s, contributed decisively to the progressive liberalisation of sexual mores. However, it is not possible to disprove absolutely and definitively those who suspect that even the cases of hysteria reported by Freud and the psychoanalysts are, as in those described by Charcot, the fruit of a construction or at least a co-construction between therapists and patients. On the other hand, Freud, after having long been idealised and treated as a hero, finally became the target of a campaign of systematic attacks (the so-called *Freud bashing*).

Freud did not define hysteria on the basis of possible florid physical symptoms, but rather in relation to particular personality characteristics. Hysteria was characterised in his eyes essentially as "unsatisfied desire", i.e. an unconscious will to remain in a desiring state. The sufferer would typically fall victim to an "Oedipus complex", whereby during childhood the person would wish to replace the parent of their own sex in order to be close to the parent of the opposite sex, but would eventually renounce this desire, having *introjected* the parental prohibitions. This means, in Freud's language, that in the person's mind a particularly punitive "superego" has built up, i.e. a psychic instance that replaces external prohibitions with internal prohibitions, the nature of which is never fully conscious. A person is led, in practice, to renew in adult life the suspended condition of childhood. A hysterical personality forbids itself sexual satisfaction by means of a series of stratagems that keep them in the condition of aspiring to something that cannot be obtained: in the field of love, they will always fall in love with the unavailable person and will always be uninterested in people who seek them.

1.3 Other Times, Other Hysterias

We have sometimes referred, for simplicity's sake, to "hysterics" as mainly female patients, even though male hysteria, although much less diagnosed, was not ignored by Charcot and Freud. However, hysteria, even when deprived of its most spectacular connotations, has generally been described – as noted above – as a kind of caricature of stereotyped female behaviour: impressionability, superficiality, fainting, hypersensitivity, and other clichés which are linked as much to the clinical description of the hysteric as, with less emphasis, to a misogynist conception of women. In any case, having lost or limited the symptom of "conversion", hysteria has continued to be diagnosed to this day by generations of psychoanalysts, who recognise both hysterical personalities *tout court* and more moderate "hysterical traits" in people who seem to sabotage their own attempts to construct an existential fulfilment, especially in the erotic sphere. Having changed customs, a hysterical person may perhaps have some sexual life, but with little satisfaction.

> Patients with hysterical personality disorder [...] usually present with problems that revolve around either genital sexuality per se or around difficulties with the sexual objects in their lives. Although the hysterical female has classically been described as "frigid", or anorgasmic, she may also be promiscuous and fully orgasmic but basically dissatisfied with her sexual relationships. She may be unable to make a romantic or sexual commitment to a man who is appropriate for her, instead falling hopelessly in love with an unavailable man. Another recurring problem for the female hysterical patient is that men often misinterpret

her actions as sexual advances, and she is continually surprised at this misunderstanding - a fact that reflects the *unconscious* nature of her seductiveness.[17].

The clinical picture of self-sabotage, of course, fits also the identification of a male hysteric, who can have varied behavioural characteristics: "The descriptions of male hysterical patients fall into two broad subtypes: the hypermasculine and the passive, effeminate".[18]

Outside of the psychoanalytic movement, however, not only conversion hysteria but also hysteria in the broader sense seems to have disappeared. Already the DSM-III, i.e. the third edition of the Diagnostic and Statistical Manual of Mental Disorders compiled by the American Psychiatric Association,[19] removed hysteria from the list of diagnosable mental illnesses. Currently, "conversion disorder" and "histrionic personality disorder" are categorised as different nosological entities.

Conversion disorder in the DSM could be described as conversion without hysteria. It consists of "one or more symptoms of altered voluntary motor or sensory function" that cannot be explained by a neurological disease or another mental illness (e.g. depression or panic attack disorder), resulting in "clinically significant distress or impairment in social, occupational, or other important areas".[20] It seems significant that in the DSM the hypothesis of a traumatic cause returns to the fore: "Onset may be associated with stress or trauma, either psychological or physical in nature. The potential etiological relevance of this stress or trauma may be suggested by a close temporal relationship".[21] Interestingly, the main risk factors are temperamental (as thought by Charcot) or environmental, specifically "a history of childhood abuse and neglect",[22] as thought by the early Freud. We are, however, dealing with a disorder considered extremely rare, diagnosed in no more than 5 cases out of 100,000 each year. Even if we were to consider conversion disorder the same nosological entity as classical hysteria at the end of the 19th century, but described perhaps more objectively, we would still have to consider it to have all but disappeared.

The histrionic personality is similar to, but not overlapping with, what has been described by psychoanalysts as the hysterical personality (epidemiological studies find very little correlation of this diagnosis with that of conversion disorder). The "style" of the histrionic person is described as seductive, but in an inadequate, boorish, primitive way, such that the desire in the other person, instead of being aroused, completely dissipates. To summarise the differences between histrionic and hysterical personalities, one can consider their respective conduct in psychotherapy. Both tend to "eroticise" the transference, i.e. to desire the therapist sexually. The hysterical personality, however, tends to understand the improper nature of their desire, whereas the histrionic personality considers sex with the professional a concrete and realisable possibility. In both cases, circumstances are well known in which the very person who was supposed to mark the inviolability of boundaries was the first to cross them.[23]

Notes

1 Breuer and Freud, *Studies on Hysteria*, 35.
2 Freud, *Autobiographical Study.*
3 Macmillan, *Freud Evaluated*; Esterson, *Seductive Mirage*; Mecacci, *Il caso Marylyn M.*
4 Corraze, "La question de l'hystérie".
5 See Sydenham, *Epistolary Dissertation.*
6 Goldstein, *Console and Classify.*
7 Freud, *The Neuro-Psychoses of Defence.*
8 Goldstein, *Console and Classify.*
9 Aragon and Breton, "Le cinquantenaire de l'hystérie".
10 Dibattista, *Charcot e il linguaggio della neurologia.*
11 Ellenberger, *The Discovery of the Unconscious.*
12 Breuer and Freud, *Studies on Hysteria*, 7
13 Plas, *Naissance d'une science humaine.*
14 Freud, *On the History*, 15.
15 Freud, *The Psychopathology of Everyday Life.*
16 Gabbard, *Psychodynamic Psychiatry*, 20.
17 Gabbard, *Psychodynamic Psychiatry*, 428.
18 Gabbard, *Psychodynamic Psychiatry*, 429.
19 After the American Psychiatric Association (APA), *Diagnostic and Statistical Manual* (*DSM*)-III, which constitutes a kind of bible of diagnosis throughout the Western world, four other editions or sub-editions came out with the acronyms *DSM*-III-R (revised), *DSM*-IV-TR (text revised), *DSM*-5, and *DSM*-5-TR. The only "competitor" to the *DSM* is the *ICD* (*International Classification of Diseases*), published by World Health Organisation, which groups all medical diagnoses, not only psychiatric ones.
20 APA, *DSM-5-TR*, 360.
21 APA, *DSM-5-TR*, 360.
22 APA, *DSM-5-TR*, 360.
23 Gabbard and Lester, *Boundaries and Boundary.*

2 Tarantism

2.1 The Story of Maria of Nardò

On 24 June 1959, a team led by the Italian anthropologist Ernesto De Martino and comprising, among others, a psychoanalyst, a doctor, and a photographer, has just arrived in Nardò, Salento, to search for evidence of a ritual that has been linked to "tarantism" for centuries: the bite of the tarantula is cured with music and dance. The team has been informed that a local man, who runs a barbershop, is also a musician in a group that performs similar rituals. Upon arriving at the shop, De Martino and his team discover they have been lucky: the barber is playing at that very moment at the home of "tarantata", i.e. a woman was bitten by a spider and suffering from *tarantism*. Guided by the echoes of the musical instruments, among which there is the obsessive rhythm of a tambourine, they find the house of the *tarantata* in the alleyways, where a group of people has gathered. They smile and explain that they are there for reasons of study, amidst the somewhat curious looks of the villagers. They manage to enter the house and find themselves "thrown into another planet". In the house, consisting of only one room and lit almost only by the light coming in through the front door, the team sees a large white sheet lying on the floor on top of blankets, where the *tarantata* is lying. All around are the musicians, images of St Peter and St Paul, a jug of "miraculous" water drawn from the well of San Paolo in Galatina, an offering basket, while the fireplace is shielded by a red cloth on which a crucifix has been hung, suggesting that Christ's blood has been shed on the wall. An acrid smell pervades the room. Both the *tarantata* and the musicians have engaged in the ritual for hours. De Martino vividly describes the scenario:

> Here, within the limits marked by the white canvas, the tarantata danced, dressed in white like the canvas on which she danced, her waist cinched by a sash, her black hair tempestuously loose and falling back over her olive-coloured face, whose ostentatiously immobile and hard features could be glimpsed, and whose eyes were now closed and now half-closed, as if sleepwalking, while the guitarist, the accordionist, the

DOI: 10.4324/9781003481249-3

tambourine player and our barber-violinist produced themselves in turn in the vibrant affair of sound therapy.[1]

The same sequence is repeated for hours. The woman, Maria, married, aged 29, is lying on the ground when the band starts playing a tarantella. As soon as she hears the music, the *tarantata* produces head movements that follow the rhythm of the tambourine in an apparently automatic way. Gradually the movement extends to the body and, rhythmically, first supine and then on all fours, the woman performs a sort of dance on the ground as if identifying herself with the spider that has bitten her. Then she gets up and performs a real dance, which goes on in an initially unrefined and then increasingly controlled manner, also performing traditional figures of the tarantella dance. All this ends after about a quarter of an hour, when the *tarantata* begins to lose her rhythm. The other women then prepare to safeguard the inevitable fall to the ground. Maria drinks and rests for about ten minutes. The musicians, having dried off their copious sweat and quenched their thirst, resume the musical initiative and the cycle continues.

At ten in the evening, the exhausted musicians put away their instruments and give the *tarantata* an appointment for ten o'clock AM the next day. A short, stocky character appears on the scene and invites everyone to leave. He is the owner of the estate where Maria works as a labourer, and he is the person who is going to pay the orchestra for the musical performance. He needs Maria to return to work as soon as possible. As long as she remains in her condition, she is unable to eat and only gets out of bed for music therapy. Maria is asked if St Paul has spoken to her, whether he has granted her "grace" to be delivered from her condition. Maria barely replies. It becomes clear that the saint has not yet intervened.

The next morning the cycle of the ritual occurs again. When she wakes up, Maria slips out of bed onto the white sheet. She continues to feel compelled to dance to the rhythm of the tarantella, but in the course of the morning, a few signs reassure the villagers that the moment of grace is near: a few shrieks, Maria's willingness to have some food. De Martino's team is informed that the saint normally releases the *tarantati* at precise times during the day: at 12, 1, 3, or 5 o'clock. Otherwise, it will be for the next day. In fact, right around three o'clock in the afternoon, Maria reports hearing a voice telling her in dialect "I give you grace". Exhausted, she lies down to rest. As a counterevidence, the little orchestra again plays a tarantella, but the woman no longer feels compelled to follow the rhythm. The next step involves a thanksgiving visit to the church in Galatina dedicated to St Paul, where Maria goes the day after her "liberation". Here she performs a casual tarantella without the accompaniment of music, drinks a glass of water from the miraculous well, and for that year at least she is free of her problems and can resume her modest work as a farmer and gleaner. Presumably, a new crisis will arise next year, as the feast of St Peter and Paul, which falls on 27 June, approaches.

At the age of 13, Maria lost her father, whom she was particularly attached to. She spent her teenage years with her mother (whom she did not really love), in the home of some relatives, where she basically starved. At the age of 18, she fell in love with a boy of her own age, but her love, although reciprocated, was hindered by his parents. A marriage would, in their opinion, have been ruled out for financial reasons. The boy left her.

Still in anguish over lost love, on a certain Sunday at noon, Maria was allegedly bitten by a tarantula. Even then she was treated with the complex ritual which was just described, but the cure is temporary. According to the story, as long as the tarantula is alive (or its progeny is alive, since the spider can transmit to them a kind of ownership of the poison inoculated into the victims), Maria falls ill every year and could not leave her bed without the intervention of the orchestra and the grace granted by St Paul. Maria is one of the last *tarantate*.

2.2 The Apulian Disease

Tarantism is a pathological condition linked, in popular belief, to the poisoning caused by the bite of a spider – the *taranta* or *tarantula* – the effects of which can be cured through a specific ritual, as seen in the story of Maria of Nardò. The ritual first of all uses specific music, codified over time, of which there are written examples as far back as the 17th century. A famous example of these is Atanasius Kircher's *Antidotum tarantulae*, which has been published several times in pre-baroque music recordings. In the popular tradition, therapeutic music is essentially based on a dance rhythm, the tarantella, which entered the festive repertoire of the South. Even Tchaikovsky, in 1880, uses a tarantella in *Capriccio Italiano*, which was the result of sound impressions from his trip to the Peninsula. In addition to music, the traditional therapy involves special sensory stimulation to induce a trance in the sufferer during which the person produces a spontaneous dance that frees them, at least temporarily, from the harmful effects of the poison. Coloured ribbons are used, for example, both to be *seen* and to be *used* in the dance. The colour of the ribbons is of particular importance, because it evokes the spider's spots, which can be different. Thus, if the spider's spots are red, it is important that there are red ribbons. To what extent the colour is appropriate can be established from the reactions of the dancer: if they follow the rhythm of the music properly, this means that the ribbons are the right ones. Moreover, according to the tradition, if the *tarantato* has been bitten close to a river or water source, containers of water must be placed where the treatment is carried out.

> The taranta, the bite, the poisoning, the music, the dance, the colours — in short 'crisis', 'cure', 'healing' — constitute a symbolic system, a cultural nexus which in its ceremonial dynamic fulfils a resolving,

rebalancing and reintegrating function of conflicts, frustrations, individual and collective traumas.[2]

The geographical location of the phenomenon of tarantism is extremely narrow. Its spread has never gone beyond the borders of the Kingdom of the two Sicilies. Specifically, tarantism has from the outset been limited almost exclusively to Apulia, eventually remaining confined to the Salento area, but excluding the "feud of Galatina", whose inhabitants, thanks to the blessings of St Paul, have always been protected from the effects of the spider's bite. St Francis as well is considered a protector, hence the Franciscan friars would themselves have been immune to tarantism.

The phenomenon of tarantism is the subject of a book that has achieved great notoriety in Italy, *The Land of Remorse (La terra del rimorso)*, by anthropologist Ernesto De Martino, who collaborated with, among others, Giovanni Jervis, one of the best-known Italian psychiatrists and psychoanalysts of the 20th century. De Martino organised a field study in Apulia in 1959, which lasted only three weeks, when very few cases had been reported. The team heard of only 37 cases (of which 33 were women). By 1974 the cases had been reduced to 16.[3] At the dawn of the new millennium, tarantism seemed to have disappeared.[4] Paradoxically, however, the folklore music created to induce dance therapy seems to be enjoying new popularity today. Events such as the "Notte della Taranta" (Night of the Taranta) attract large audiences and even well-known personalities such as Stewart Copeland, former drummer of the Police, who has participated in the event several times.

The phenomenon is very old. It has fascinated various scholars over the centuries, showing, as the following section will illustrate, further antecedents and parallels in Europe. Although paradoxical effects of spider bites were repeatedly reported in southern Italy between the 11th and 16th centuries, the first mentions of the related music therapy date back to the 14th century, and the first hints of dance in the mid-16th century.

The first document attesting to the positive effects of music on the tarantula's bite would be, according to Ernesto De Martino,[5] the *Sertum papale de venenis* (Decree of the Pope on venoms), an ecclesiastical manuscript dedicated to remedies for poisoning. However, in this text, the cure appears to be linked to the improvement of the affected person's mood. The tarantula's bite would induce a melancholic condition in the tarantula sufferer, which cheerful music could lift (the "tarantella" is already mentioned here as a possible example of suitable music). De Martino also enlists the book *De venenis* (On venoms) by Cristoforo degli Onesti, a professor of medicine in Padua towards the end of the 14th century. Here, in the index of the manuscript, there appears a chapter on the bite of the tarantula, which has unfortunately been lost.

In 1548, Ortensio Lando and Piero Andrea Mattioli independently mentioned the curative effects of dancing on the tarantula bite, although only the former of the two ruled out other remedies having an effect. A letter from 1590 written by Antonio Maria Manzoli, Bishop of Gravina, and addressed to the naturalist Ulisse Aldrovandi is perhaps the first specific report on the issue.[6] Manzoli wrote: "The man bitten [by the tarantula] is very troubled and especially in the parts of the heart, and in a moment, he becomes so hungry that he loses his appetite and becomes very weak". Sure signs that he is tarantula-ridden are inappetence and a real phobia towards meat. The remedy is then only one: not doctors and medicines that "make you worse", but "certain *sonatori*" ("musicians") who start rehearsing various pieces of music. The *tarantato* does not move until he hears the tone that suits his poison. Then he rises from his bed and "immediately becomes like a lion, for by such a sound his strength and colour return to him, and he begins to jump and dance with such strength and speed that he amazes everyone".[7]

Manzoli is also the first author to mention three different animals as possible causes of an otherwise similar pathology: the tarantula, the "solfrizzo", and the scorpion.[8] According to the tradition, very similar effects can be induced by the actual tarantula (*Lycosa tarentula*), by a spider resembling the black widow spider, but less dangerous, which presumably corresponds to Manzoli's "solfrizzo" (*Latrodectus tredecimguttatus*), by the scorpion or even by a snake, the effects of which can be felt even if it is only seen near a water course. In fact, the Apulian tarantula is a spider whose bite is painful but brings no particular consequences. High fever, convulsions, insomnia, and abdominal pains (which disappear after a couple of days, except in rare cases of complications) are produced instead by the neurotoxic venom of the *Latrodectus*, which, however, does not cause immediate pain. If one considers that the *Latrodectus* is less visible and hides in walls, while the tarantula is larger and lives in the fields, it is possible to imagine that in several cases farmers may have attributed to an innocent tarantula the effects of the bite of the more devious local black widow.[9] Certainly, the actual symptoms induced by the *Latrodectus* do not, as is quite obvious, constitute a direct physiological reason for the condition of the *tarantato*. However, it is quite understandable how these symptoms and their relatively rapid disappearance may have been absorbed and reworked in a "symbolic order" – to use De Martino's words – which generated the cultural beliefs about tarantism and its suggestions.

> The intermittent tremor that is localised mainly in the lower limbs, and which can sometimes take on a convulsive aspect, is interpreted as a hint of dance, which must develop in order to allow the evil to express itself and to come out into the open through a full realisation of these movements, namely dance.[10]

When Manzoli wrote to Aldrovandi, the phenomenon was already known outside the borders of the Kingdom of Naples. Baldassarre Castiglione mentioned it in *The Book of the Courtier (Il libro del Cortegiano)* and Jean Bodin in the *Republique*. Cesare Ripa, in his *Iconologia*, perhaps the largest repertoire of allegorical images ever published, seemed to identify *tarantismo* as a symbol par excellence of Apulia. The region was in fact represented as follows: "A woman of fair complexion, who, clothed in a thin veil, has tarantulas on her [...] and is in the act of dancing".[11] Ripa specifies:

> The tarantulas, stained with different colours, are represented as animals that are very well known and unique in this province, as well as to demonstrate [...] the diversity of their venom, because when they bite someone, different and strange things happen: some sing, some laugh, some cry, some shout, some sleep, some wake, some jump, some tremble, some sweat, and some suffer other different things, and they go crazy as if they were spirits.[12]

The book *Iconologia* seems to be the first source to mention the importance of colours in therapy.[13] In the 17th century, tarantism, no longer a mere local curiosity, began to be studied more carefully from both a medical and a religious perspective. Some monographs on the subject received considerable attention, even internationally: in particular those by Ferdinando Epifanio[14] and Giorgio Baglivi.[15] Epifanio did not have any doubt on the veracity of the symptoms, nor the efficacy of the dancing cure: "qui nobis non crediet, veniet, et videat" ("whoever does not believe in us come and see for yourself").[16] Baglivi reported just a few perplexities from the medical world, which however he took care to refute, proving convincing even for an English author of some renown (R. Mead), who mentions tarantism in his medical work.[17] Baglivi, however, having conducted some sort of field research, became convinced that not all the alleged *tarantati* had actually been bitten.

> He devised the distinction between two tarantisms, the 'real' one caused by the bite of the *taranta*, and the 'fake' one from which the *mulierculae* [little women] profited to celebrate their *carnivals*. This distinction later became normative in order to settle in the medical perspective what resisted the reduction of tarantism to a disease. The rest that resulted from the reduction was polemically devalued as 'false' and 'fake' tarantism, as fanaticism and superstition.[18]

Tarantism was eventually Christianised. Linked as it was to a pagan ritual, it was initially viewed with a hostile, but all in all uninterested, attitude by the Church. From the local bishops came *ex officio* condemnations that seemed dictated more by a desire to avoid accusations of complete neglect on the subject. Instead, it was the Jesuits, who considered the South a sort of Italian India to be evangelised, who tackled the issue head-on. Using a technique of *accommodation to the capacities of the people*, the Jesuits did not even try to eradicate popular beliefs but superimposed the cult of saints on them during the 18th century.[19] Thus the idea of St Paul's protection was born, with the consequent possibility of asking him as a grace for an at least temporary end to the torments of tarantism and immunity from the effects of the spider bite for the Galatina area, of which the saint had become patron. Moreover, the replacement of pagan beliefs with Christian beliefs, of ancient gods with saints, of temples with churches, was certainly not unique to Apulia but rather constituted the rule in the history of the spread of Christianity. Even Christmas and Easter are the heritage of Neolithic festivals: that of the sprouting of grain and that of the harvest.

It was not until the 18th century that someone seriously began to question, in a scientific context, the veracity of the accounts of tarantism. Francesco Serao even tried to ridicule the beliefs about the effects of the tarantula bite and the need for dance therapy.[20] Serao was an interpreter of a new cultural temperament in the Kingdom of Naples, which had first absorbed the lessons of scepticism and the new philosophical-scientific culture of 17th-century Europe (Bacon, Gassendi, Hobbes, Descartes) and then became part of the Enlightenment strand, thus standing in direct contrast to the Jesuit Catholic approach. Serao started from an in-depth study of pre-existing material, but above all from an extensive collection of data provided by local correspondents and actual experiments on the effects of the arachnid bite.

> On the basis of these considerations, Serao concluded that the cause of tarantism was not to be found in the tarantula but in the Apulians [...] whom Valletta had already portrayed as impatient to stand still and therefore in need of dissolving with music and dance 'a certain intestine seriousness or oppression', a melancholy which reigned in these lands. When they were subject to evils, in extreme moments, the Apulians resorted to the institution of tarantism, heir to the ancient orgiastic cults.[21]

Serao's text was enormously popular among southern Italian *literati* and doctors, to the point of convincing them that its publication alone could cause the phenomenon to progressively decline until it disappeared. Which in reality did not happen, since for at least another century and a half its widespread diffusion is attested. This does not seem at all incomprehensible, given that the culture into which tarantism is grafted is that of the "peasant" environment, steeped in magical beliefs and completely impermeable to possible "cultured" influences. This is a 20th-century description of this phenomenon:

> *Tarantati* are people who do not present any precise psychic illness, but a number of disorders caused by various social, economic and cultural frustrations. In order to understand and frame this phenomenon in its proper light, the real and miserable living conditions in which the southern peasant is forced to live must be taken into account. Deprived

> as they are of any means of being able to plan their own life, they are the victim of an unbearable situation of abandonment: they know nothing but deprivation, sacrifice, and in many cases hunger: shrines, patron saints and, as their only solution and hope, emigration, which will lead them to survive by becoming a slave to some foreign industry.[22]

The idea of a connection between the orgiastic cults of Dionysus and tarantism proposed by Serao was later taken up by Domenico Solito[23] and adopted as a key interpretation by Henry Sigerist.[24] The latter believed that, at least originally, the alleged *tarantati* simulated having been bitten by an animal only to be able to continue practising pagan rites that the Church would not tolerate. However, there seems to be no trace of an underground history of such rites between the twilight of ancient paganism and the Middle Ages. In any case, the Apulian *tarantati* observed by De Martino and Jervis seemed anything but simulators. It seemed much more likely that they had a real, deep conviction that they had been bitten by the tarantula and experienced a conversion of psychological problems into somatic symptoms, as it had happened to the hysterics observed by Charcot and Freud: a conversion oriented by cultural beliefs, suggested by a particular environment.

2.3 Pathology, Music, Dance, and Therapy

The belief that it is possible to cure various pathological conditions with music is very ancient and attested in many cultures. Suffice it to say that in the *Book of Samuel* (16:14–23), it is reported that David was called upon to heal King Saul, who was being persecuted by an evil spirit (which, according to some biblical philologists, corresponded to a melancholic condition), with his zither; or that shamanic rituals have always involved a musical trance.[25]

On the contrary, the identification of a pathology characterised by a "dancing mania" seemed to have a late medieval origin. A chronicle from 1021 "describes the dancing of eighteen villagers at the church of the monastery of Kolbig (Bernburg), who were condemned by the priest Luperto to continue dancing and shouting for a whole year".[26] Various historical accounts testify that in July 1374, in various cities along the banks of the Rhine and Moselle rivers, various people threw themselves into frenzied dancing in the town squares, hurling unconscious cries that to some seemed demonic invocations. The forced dancers seemed to become furious at certain colours (especially red) and particular objects (such as clogs); in any case, they continued dancing until they were exhausted, when they let themselves fall to the ground inert. Similar cases occurred within a few months in Liège, Aix-la Chapelle, Cologne, and Metz.

The contagion spread rapidly to hundreds of people. Since, under the pretext of the epidemic, groups of people took to moving from town to town and exploiting the alleged pathological condition to commit theft and other crimes, there was a harsh repression of the maniacs by the authorities, which caused the dancing mania to disappear from 1380 onwards for thirty years. However, a new manifestation of the phenomenon occurred in 1418, starting in the city of Strasbourg, where the expression "St Vitus' dance" was coined.[27] The 16th century witnessed, especially in the German-speaking area, a kind of epidemic of what doctors began to classify as *Viti saltus*. Its origin is generally considered magical and demonic, and against it, the protection of St Vitus takes on the role that St Paul will acquire in Apulia.

> St Vitus's chapels in various parts of Europe, especially the one in the southern German city of Ulm, become a place of pilgrimage and bands of dancers stricken by *Veitstanz* every year gather, men and women, around the chapel of St Vitus and driven by a common, collective abandon they form circles, hand in hand, dancing day and night in a mad delirium until they fall to the ground exhausted. During these violent leaps, they are seized by visions and hallucinations, and call aloud to the spirits. Some of them tell of feeling immersed in a river of blood that forced them to jump to get out [...] After engaging in this wild dance near the chapel, many are cured thanks to the saint's intercession, returning home in good spirits and with a sure footing.[28]

The parallels between the two pathologies are therefore multiple: in both cases, there is first and foremost a compulsion to dance that is fostered by music and the protection of a saint. There is also an illustrious iconographic example for the dance of St Vitus: a drawing by Bruegel the Elder from 1564, preserved in the Albertina Museum in Vienna. It depicts figures in the throes of St Vitus' dance, stimulated to dance by bagpipe players. For some time, however, the expression "St Vitus' dance" has become synonymous with an organic disease known as "Sydenham Chorea". The miraculous healing of Diocletian's son (subject to compulsive movements of presumably epileptic origin) has been attributed to St Vitus, who would then paradoxically repay the Saint with martyrdom for refusing to pay homage to the pagan gods. The disappearance of the illness linked to the alleged dance compulsion did not, however, prevent the birth of a piece of music that has enjoyed a certain notoriety, entitled "Il ballo di San Vito" ("St Vitus' Dance"), written by the Italian composer Vinicio Capossela.

Finally, it was Ernesto De Martino himself who pointed out the affinity of tarantism with Sardinian *àrgia*, in which a male person would be bitten by the soul of a female dead person.[29] The bite would cause the transmigration of the soul of the dead person into the living, leading to different conduct in the case of the possessing soul belonging to a maiden, a bride (usually pregnant), or a widow. In the former case, the therapeutic ritual employs dance and music, as in tarantism: the possessed person chooses a dancer with whom to dance repeatedly until exhaustion. The bride's spirit is appeased with a symbolic delivery and suckling with the help of a puppet. That of the widow is accompanied by a funeral lament for her dead husband by a choir.[30]

For further considerations regarding possession, however, it will be appropriate to refer to the next chapter.

Notes

1 De Martino, *La terra del rimorso*, 87.
2 Turchini, *Morso, morbo, morte*, 15.
3 Montinaro, *Salento povero*.
4 Palmisano, "Presenza, Assenza e Rappresentazione".
5 De Martino, *La terra del rimorso*.
6 Turchini, *Morso, morbo, morte*.
7 Manzoli, "La più antica relazione sulla tarantola", 201.
8 Manzoli, "La più antica relazione sulla tarantola", 202.
9 Pepe, Panzera, and Durante, "Il tarantismo: i responsabili".
10 Fantini, "Il tarantismo e il ballo di San Vito", 76.
11 Ripa, *Iconologia*, 320.
12 Ripa, *Iconologia*, 321.
13 Cazzato, "La Taranta Filologa".
14 Epiphanius, *Centum Historiae*.
15 Baglivi, "De anatome morsu".
16 Epiphanius, *Centum historiae*, 261.
17 See Cazzato, "La taranta filologa".
18 De Martino, *La terra del rimorso*, 272.
19 Spedicato, "Chiesa e trasgressione".
20 Serao, *Della tarantola*.
21 De Martino, *La terra del rimorso*, 278-279.
22 Rossi, *Lettere da una tarantata*, 8.
23 Solito, *Descrizione Storico-filosofica*.
24 Sigerist, "The Story of Tarantism".
25 Rouget, *Music and Trance*.
26 Di Lecce, "Delle tarantole", 87.
27 Fantini, "Il tarantismo e il ballo di San Vito".
28 Fantini, "Il tarantismo e il ballo di San Vito", 70.
29 De Martino, *La terra del rimorso*.
30 Gallini, *I rituali dell'árgia*.

3 Demonic Possession

3.1 The Story of Anneliese

Anneliese Michel was a Catholic and traditionalist girl from a Catholic and traditionalist family in Klingenberg, a village near Munich, an environment in which being Catholic and traditionalist was no exception. In the mid-1970s, Anneliese began to have visions. Menacing faces suddenly appeared to her. The symptoms were interpreted by doctors as the expression of an epileptic focus in the left temporal region. Neither the girl nor her parents, however, really believed in the physical diagnosis. Instead, Anneliese was convinced that she was possessed by a demon and, with the support of her family, decided to turn to the Church for exorcism. Once permission had been obtained from the Church authorities, local priests began a series of exorcism rites starting in September 1975.

From that moment on, the visions increased rather than decreasing. The girl became convinced that she was possessed not by one but by six different entities. Of these, only one was identifiable as an actual demon. It was indeed the devil, Lucifer himself. The other five "possessors" corresponded to deceased human beings, particularly disliked in Anneliese's environment. They were a locally known priest, named Fleischmann, and four much more famous characters: Cain, Judas, Nero, and Hitler. During the visions, Anneliese gave voice to the six characters, but they did not express hatred towards the world around them, as anyone who has seen films such as *The Exorcist* (which, incidentally, had been released shortly before, in 1973) would expect. On the contrary, Lucifer and co. complained about the apparent abandonment of traditional Catholic values in the world around them. One of their favourite targets was Hans Küng, a theologian who was also well-known abroad for some time. Küng was a fervent advocate of inter-religious dialogue and the abolition of priestly celibacy and also a severe critic of the dogma of papal infallibility.

Anneliese Michel gradually became convinced that she was destined for sacrifice. Through her death, she would help redeem the Catholic world, which had accepted principles (those of the Second Vatican Council) that went against tradition. And death finally came on 1 July 1976, after Anneliese

DOI: 10.4324/9781003481249-4

had subjected herself to fasting and self-flagellation, without the comfort of medicine but only that of exorcist rites. The first consequence of her death was the most logical one in a now secularised world: the family and the priests, who shared Anneliese's value system and had kept her away from necessary medical care, were convicted of murder.

Popular religiosity, however, was not definitively convinced of the "earthly" nature of Anneliese's illness. Paradoxically, she was considered by some to be a possible saint, to the point that it was decided to exhume her body to see if it had been preserved from corruption (a circumstance that would have endorsed the idea of sanctity). Obviously, the exhumation did not show the world a miraculously incorrupt body. In any case, although the Michel case originally dealt a serious blow to the credibility of certain beliefs (it was the last exorcism attempted in Bavaria), in more recent times various Catholic authors have published contributions aimed at proving that it was a *real* possession. Some might consider them isolated cases of diehard fanatics. Not so. Today there is a resurgence of the belief that demonic possession is a real possibility in this world and that therefore exorcists are no longer folkloristic figures, but legitimate performers of rites aimed at driving real demons out of the bodies of human beings. After all, the International Association of Exorcists, originally founded by a number of priests that could be counted on the fingers of one hand, now includes hundreds of adherents and has been officially recognised since 2015 by Pope Francis. In the remainder of the chapter, an attempt will be made to answer various related questions. One could comment: "But who would undergo an exorcism?" Perhaps the reader does not remember, but if they have been baptised, they have also been exorcised.

The belief that the devil was pervasively present on earth led the early Church not only to exorcise the possessed but also to introduce an exorcism within the baptismal rite. This *preventive* exorcism, through which the baptised person immediately renounces Satan, has remained an integral part of the sacrament of Baptism. Consequently, it can be said that almost the entire Italian population, for example, has been exorcised. There is no doubt, of course, that baptismal exorcism is experienced without particular concern on the part of the parents and godfather of the baptised (who follow the rite closely) and on the part of those who officiate at the rite.

True exorcisms, however, constitute more than a formal rite, because they are performed in the conviction that the person being exorcised is truly possessed. It should immediately be noted that the Church's attitude both with regard to the reality and spread of demonic possession and, consequently, to the applicability of exorcism, has undergone considerable changes over the course of time. Generally speaking, one can observe a stable belief in the presence of possessing demons on earth throughout the first millennium and a half of Christianity's history, followed by a slow but steady and progressive decline in the following centuries and a certain counter-trend in the last few decades of our history.

3.2 Demonic Possession across Time and Space

The idea that a human being is subject to possession by a demon, or a spirit (or even an "object-sickness") is of course not solely linked to the Christian-Catholic world. This is a widespread belief, throughout the ages and across cultures. Practically all histories of psychiatry devote a more or less extensive section to these themes, assuming: (a) that possession constitutes a form of psychopathology; (b) that the rites of expulsion of the demon or possessing spirit represent a primitive form of psychotherapy, based on the attribution to the officiant of particular qualities (through the so-called *transference*) and on the influence obtained through the rites.

In fact, ritual performances have often shown a certain curative efficacy, so that the "symptoms" related to the alleged possession disappeared after the intervention of those who officiated at them. Not infrequently happened that priests and shamans also cured physical illnesses. Even this, however, does not surprise historians and researchers, because our culture has long been familiar with the so-called *placebo effect*. If a person is convinced that he or she has taken a drug that is effective against a certain illness or certain symptoms, at least in a certain number of cases the healing of the illness or the remission of symptoms occurs. This is why, when testing a new drug, it is necessary to divide the experimental group into two subgroups: one of them is to take the actual drug and the other an inactive drug (the placebo), but with the same physical appearance as the former. Only if there is a significant difference in effects between the two subgroups can the experimental drug be said to be effective.

Possession, however, presents itself in different ways across time and space and has not always been considered a condition of illness or at least a condition of danger. In Western culture, the relationship with a demon has in some cases even been taken as a privilege. The priestesses of Apollo at Delphi communed with the god to offer their oracles, and the same happened to the sibyls in Ancient Rome. *Manìa* (madness) and *mantikè* (divination) are terms that have the same etymological root *man*.[1] In Greece, the term *daimon* was used to mean both "character" and "demon", and it is well known that Socrates declared that he was incessantly urged by a demon (*daimonion*) not to engage in politics and rather to fulfil his educational mission towards the young Athenians.[2]

In other cases, possession is sought essentially and voluntarily by shamanic figures, through rituals mainly centred on music and chanting. Being possessed in this case requires a vocation and great commitment.[3] In fact, while exorcism has been practised to drive away the malefic possessed entity, special techniques have been used for the opposite purpose of attracting the presence of possessing spirits of a positive character. For the combination of these techniques, the name *adorcism* has been proposed.[4] It should also be noted that the possession trance induced by adorcism, although attempts have been made to define it univocally,[5] is considered the expression of a "wide range of problems, conflicts, and registers that converge therein"[6] and is therefore a fluid phenomenon, at least as fluid as the religious movements (even those of recent formation) that resort to it.

In some cultures, moreover, possession can take intermediate forms, which are not easy to classify. The DSM-IV-TR mentioned the presence, in North Africa and the Middle East, of a form of possession known as *zar*,[7] which was then strangely dropped from the glossary of culturally bound syndromes in the DSM-5.[8] In the *zar* and in some other declinations of the possession phenomenon in Africa described by anthropologists, such as *hori*, *sheitani*, *ngoma*, *hauka*, *mhondoro*, and *zima*,[9] possession can in fact present itself as a condition with which it is possible (at least in one's own cultural context) to coexist without too many problems.[10] In fact, the DSM-IV-TR reported:

> [In the *zar*] Persons possessed by a spirit may experience dissociative episodes that may include shouting, laughing, hitting the head against a wall, singing, or weeping. Individuals may show apathy and withdrawal, refusing to eat or carry out daily tasks, or may develop a long-term relationship with the possessing spirit. Such behaviour is not considered pathological locally.[11]

In fact, until the 18th century, there was little difference between the Christian cultural context and the rest of the world in terms of beliefs about the reality of possession. In the total absence of real scientific medicine, which did not come into being until the first half of the 19th century, the idea that invisible personal entities (whether demons, spirits, or *djinn*) could enter the bodies of human beings and cause physical and spiritual harm could still find credence.

In the history of Christianity, the problem of possession had far from marginal theological importance from the very beginning. Acts that can be interpreted as exorcisms are attributed to Jesus in the Gospels.[12] Also in the Gospels, it is attested that Jesus conferred the power to free the possessed first on the apostles[13] and later on believers in general.[14] Some ancient sources attribute the success of Christianity precisely to the established ability of believers to cast out demons. St Paul seems to have been particularly active in this field.[15]

In the very first centuries of Christianity's existence, the faculty to perform exorcisms was not reserved to persons with a particular role. The existence of exorcists occupying a specific position in the ecclesiastical hierarchy is only attested from the 3rd century onwards (in a letter from Pope Cornelius to Fabius of Antioch).[16] The first specific ordination of exorcists was instead established at the Council of Carthage in 398. In any case, no one doubted for many centuries that there was a need for exorcisms, nor of the influence of Satan, defined by the scriptures as the Adversary and the Prince of this world. Theology could discuss at most how his influence was exerted.

For instance, there was not even close agreement on the number of existing demons. It ranged from one demon, i.e. Satan himself (mono-demonism), to 133,396,668 (calculation by a bishop of Tusculum around 1400). Or they discussed the possibility of their mating, which presumably could use human dreams as a vehicle: a distinction was then made between *incubi*, active demons, and *succubi*, passive demons.

The first turning point in the Christian attitude towards the devil and demons can be traced back to the period from the end of the 16th to the beginning of the 17th century. The centuries of witch hunts had seen such a large number of people suspected of contact with demonic entities that many authors thought that a criterion had to be found to distinguish at least between certain and uncertain cases of possession. It was the Jesuit Petrus (Peter) Thyraeus (1546–1601) who was the first to deflate from the list of possible signs of possession a dozen symptoms previously considered as sure indications. It seems noteworthy that the occasion for such a significant breakthrough was the book *Loca infesta* (issued 1598), dedicated to the examination of places where a strong risk of demonic presence was to be identified.[17] The precise instructions contained in the *Rituale Romanum*, published at the instigation of Pope Paul V (issued 1614), constituted the first factual occasion for the Catholic Church to define and limit cases for the practice of exorcism.[18]

The 18th century saw in Johann Solomo Semler (1725–1791) the first Christian theologian to doubt the existence of the devil: the founder of Lutheran theological rationalism inspired an attitude in Protestant circles towards the abandonment of exorcism, which long preceded the Catholic one and did not see any more regressive movements. A real turning point, however, was the unique dispute between the Catholic priest Johann Joseph Gassner (1727–1779) and the freethinker Franz Anton Mesmer (1754–1815). Gassner also cured physical illnesses through exorcism, proving in his opinion that every ailment was the result of possession. Mesmer proved to achieve the same results with a technique he called *magnetism*. He was in fact convinced of something equally bizarre: that illnesses resulted from an alteration of the magnetic fluid that passes through every living being. Indeed, a commission charged with investigating the reality of the phenomena described by Mesmer (a commission of which Benjamin Franklin was also a member) quickly dismissed his ideas as being just as unfounded as Gassner's. Mesmer's findings, however, convinced many that certain phenomena considered "spiritual" by Gassner and many others before him should be brought back into the realm of the natural sciences and studied as such.[19]

Mesmer's experiences, however, opened a season of empirical research that eventually led to the discovery of hypnosis and suggestion. These became important tools at the dawn of the history of psychotherapy. At the same time, they helped to undermine the Christian belief that the devil's presence on earth was as continuous as had been believed in the past; but also that people who were convinced they were possessed were all actually prey to demons. A decisive shake-up was certainly inflicted by French psychiatric research, which revealed how apparent possessions were linked to delusions, i.e. pathological beliefs. In early 20th-century Catholic texts, one could already read a caution that would have been impossible a few decades earlier. It is found, for instance, in an *Ecclesiastical Lexicon* published in 1902, under the heading "exorcism":

> The Catholics and the old Lutherans [sic!] continue to use it, but very rarely, because advanced medical science has reduced to very few the diseases that are not proven to be products of purely natural causes. Hence demonology, if it is not, as some imprudently want, placed even in the aberrations of the human spirit, is a science that now refers to the study and treatment of very rare cases.[20]

In other words, one could not theoretically demolish the possibility of possession, but one had to be extremely cautious in its practical verification. In a *Dictionary of Catholic Theology*, published in France a few years later, it was admitted that the practice of exorcism had given rise to abuses, also linked to superstitious beliefs, but it was emphasised that the abuse did not in itself constitute proof of the falsity of the underlying theological idea; and a theory was even sketched out that would explain why true possessions were far less widespread in the present than in earlier times.

> The Church has not abandoned and there is no reason why it should ever abandon the practice of exorcisms; even exorcisms in the full and primitive sense of the term, that is, rites designed to expel the devil from persons, places or objects where his presence and his influence is betrayed through sensible manifestations. But it is a traditional doctrine, already formulated by St Hilary and St Alphonsus [...] that with the universal spread of Christianity the devil has seen his power diminished and that consequently cases of actual possession have become much rarer.[21]

In the following decades, there was a progressive tendency within the Catholic Church to put exorcism and possession into oblivion. In the 1917 *Code of Canon Law*, it was stipulated that an exorcism should only be practised after formal authorisation by a bishop, which could only be granted to priests of the highest reputation, capable of judging the plausibility of the possession.[22] In later years, provincial and diocesan statutes tended to neglect the instructions on the conduct of exorcists that had previously been omnipresent and detailed.[23] A Catholic author explained this circumstance at the time by a greater critical sense on the part of the ecclesiastical hierarchies, by a better fine-tuning of the theological doctrine explaining the degrees and modalities of Satan's intervention in the world, but also by progress in the knowledge of mental illness.[24] From the 1930s–1940s, Catholic psychiatrists also recounted cases of pseudo-possession.[25] At this point in time, only *two* phenomena could be considered definite signs of demonic possession: *xenoglossia* (the possessed person spoke languages unknown to him or herself) and a display of strength beyond that possible under normal circumstances.[26]

Some theologians, especially after the Second Vatican Council, even began to propose the idea that the devil, rather than a real and personal entity, should be regarded as a symbol of evil.[27] This was never the official opinion of the Church,[28] but before the advent of John Paul II lay observers tended to record a real disappearance of interest in the devil on the Catholic side.[29]

The advent of Pope Wojtila, however, proved decisive for a complete turn-around. The clearest proof of his convictions is a speech given on 13 August 1986 during a papal audience, almost entirely devoted to the devil's presence and action on humanity. Karol Wojtila insisted that the very building of the Kingdom of Heaven was "always exposed to the threats of the Evil One". Woe to those who underestimated its power, which extended to the entire universe! Those who denied the devil's existence showed that they were directly under his influence and became an instrument of his strategy: hiding themselves in order to better achieve his ends. Undeniable was the fact that this enormous influence on Earth also led to possessions by demons in his service. Wojtila was not only convinced that the devil was active on earth, but he himself officiated at exorcisms in the Vatican and, as a significant symbolic act, on 24 April 1988 he beatified Francisco Palau (1811–1872), a priest who had opened an institute for the mentally ill in which the admission protocol required a preliminary exorcism: those who were cured by the exorcism were evidently possessed, while the others would be hospitalised normally.

It was a very dangerous procedure, because it risked reinforcing any possible psychotic delirium of possession, as Catholic psychiatry itself has recognised for some time.[30] It could be noted that, even from a theological point of view, the protocol was wrong: exorcism is technically a *sacramental* and not a *sacrament*. The difference between the two rites is that while the latter obtains the required grace *ex opere operato* (i.e. by the very fact of being performed), the former is not always efficacious. This means that, according to Catholic doctrine, exorcism does not necessarily drive out the demon (which explains, incidentally, the priests' insistence with Anneliese). Therefore, if we place ourselves in the doctrinal perspective, Palau could not have ruled out the possibility that the patients he exorcised without result were actually possessed!

In any case, Palau was a character who saw demons everywhere. He was treated with extreme coldness by the Church of his time, which supported the secular authorities when they had him arrested, suspecting that the institution he created did not care at all about the mental health of in-patients.

Pope Wojtila was also a proponent of collaboration between faith and science in every field, including psychiatry and psychology, which initiated a process that led to the founding of the Italian Association of Catholic

Psychiatrists and Psychologists. The latter's first conference dealt with the subject of possession, going so far as to propose a *differential diagnosis* between true and false possession and bringing the subject back from theology to science. The result of this process is truly paradoxical. If at the beginning of the 20th century, the idea of demonic possession had practically disappeared from the West, at the dawn of the New Millennium dozens and dozens of people have turned to the exorcist. The number of exorcists multiplied incredibly, especially in Italy and Poland (the countries where Wojtila's influence was naturally felt most). When it was established, the International Association of Exorcists that we mentioned earlier counted five people, practically all those left in the world to practise the rite. Today, more than 300 exorcists are active in Italy alone (figure taken from the Association's website).[31] There is no reliable census of possession cases, but such an exponential increase in the number of people officiating at exorcism suggests that the estimate of thousands in Italy alone is reliable.

Just as at one time a hypothesis was formulated for the decrease in the presence of demons in the bodies of human beings, there are those who have attempted to explain the reasons why there would be such a resurgence of the phenomenon today. Two in particular would be the reasons for the return of the devil on earth: the practice of Satanism, which would be increasingly widespread, and the now dramatic affirmation of rock music (in particular the metal genre), which would convey demonic messages.[32] The expansion of the fashion for tattoos could also be an important reason, since getting a tattoo would in itself be a way to get closer to Satan, at least according to the most media-savvy of the exorcists, namely, Father Amorth.[33]

Let us pretend for a moment that we take such claims seriously: it would be complicated to explain why Italian metal fans or Polish tattooists should act as the most effective virtual antenna to attract demons to their territory. Not to mention Satanists, who are in fact a phenomenon reduced to a few dozen in Italy as elsewhere: a phenomenon generally considered folkloristic and inoffensive even by law enforcement agencies, except for sensational but entirely isolated cases such as that of the "Beasts of Satan" in Italy, guilty of four murders at the turn of the century; or the Manson followers in the United States, responsible for the murder of Sharon Tate, which inspired Quentin Tarantino's *Once Upon a Time in Hollywood*.

3.3 True Possession

The paradox of today's situation is related to the possibility of using an alleged scientific lens to exclude a psychiatric diagnosis. Catholic psychiatrists and psychologists, led in Italy by Professor Tonino Cantelmi, share the basic principle that great caution is needed to distinguish various conditions that might wrongly be considered diabolic signs from "true" possession. An untrained psychologist might consider entirely human phenomena such as delusions, panic attacks, obsessions, and compulsions as signs of supernatural presence.[34] Other signs, symptoms, and phenomena that might lead one to suspect demonic intervention, although numerous and varied, remain uncertain.[35] There are three symptoms, however, that are considered by these observers an almost sure indication of diabolic infestation: dual personality, paranormal phenomena, and phenomena that are, to use the authors' words, "different or contrary to scientific methods".[36] In essence, these are the same principles of differential diagnosis as previously set out by an exorcist, namely, Father Balducci, whose words Cantelmi's group reuses almost exactly.[37]

However, do paranormal phenomena exist? Are there really phenomena that are "different or contrary" to science? No person belonging to any scientific community has ever observed any. The best known of these alleged paranormal phenomena, the act of speaking unknown languages, is usually explained by the suggestion induced by the babbling of the allegedly possessed person, who occasionally recalls the sound of authentic words in an unknown language, or one barely heard by observers (as may be the case of Aramaic by a priest, who at one time studied theology). The alleged Herculean power of the possessed is a condition well known to nurses who find themselves in the position of having to stop agitated psychiatric patients without causing them physical harm. Levitation has so far not been observed by witnesses considered reliable.

On the other hand, the case of split personality is an entirely human pathological form and can be explained in quite different terms than the presence of a demon. We are therefore faced with a situation in which there is a clear division between those who believe in the authenticity of at least a fair number of cases of possession and those (secular science) who consider them to be the result of religious delusions, in which, however, third parties are involved. Once upon a time, this would have been called *folie à deux* ("madness of two") or *folie à plusieurs* ("madness of many").

If, however, it is a condition linked to a form of delirium, the possessed person suffers from a real problem, the nature of which is – from a secular scientific point of view – misrepresented in a particular context. We could therefore define possession, in today's West, as the labelling as a supernatural phenomenon of a psychotic condition by a particular sub-culture, which we would be cautious to define as Catholic, because we doubt that all Catholics are willing to believe that there can be possessed people, at least in the present day (regardless of the opinion of a possibly relevant part of the ecclesiastical hierarchies).

Notes

1 Liddell and Scott, *A Greek-English Lexicon.*
2 See, e.g., Plato, *Apology of Socrates*, 31c-d, pp. 79–80.
3 See, e.g., Rouget, *Music and Trance.*
4 De Heusch, *Why Marry Her?*
5 Rouget, *Music and Trance.*

6 Beneduce, *Trance e possessione in Africa*, 72.
7 APA, *DSM-IV-TR*.
8 APA, *DSM-5*.
9 Boddy, "Spirit Possession Revisited".
10 Lewis, *Ecstatic Religion*.
11 APA, *DSM-IV-TR*, 903.
12 Mt 12. 22–30; Ma 3. 22–27; Lu 11. 14–26.
13 Mt 10.1; Ma 6.7; Lu 9.1.
14 Mt 17.20; Ma 9.28.
15 Acts 16.16-18; 19.12
16 *Patr. Lat.* III, coll. 768.
17 Thyraeus, *Loca infesta*.
18 *Rituale Romanum*.
19 Midelfort, *Exorcism and Enlightenment*.
20 Barbavara, "Esorcismo", 227.
21 Forget, "Exorcisme", 1775.
22 Peters (ed.), *Code of Canon Law*.
23 Philippeau, "Exorcisme".
24 Philippeau, "Exorcisme", 945.
25 Tonquedec, "Les maladies nerveuses", "L'action de Satan dans le monde"; Lhermitte, "Les Psudo-Possessions Diaboliques".
26 Marquart, "L'exorciste".
27 See, e.g., Kelly, *Towards the Death of Satan*.
28 See, Paul VI, *Insegnamenti*.
29 Kolakowski, "Diavolo".
30 See, e.g., Tonquedec, "Les Maladies Nerveuses".
31 https://www.agensir.it/chiesa/.
32 Cantelmi, Laselva, and Paluzzi, *Psicologia e teologia in dialogo*.
33 Amorth, *Esorcisti e psichiatri*.
34 Cantelmi, Laselva, and Paluzzi, *Psicologia e teologia in dialogo*, 77–79.
35 Cantelmi, Laselva, and Paluzzi, *Psicologia e teologia in dialogo*, 75–76.
36 Cantelmi, Laselva, and Paluzzi, *Psicologia e teologia in dialogo*, 79.
37 Balducci, *Il diavolo*; Balducci, "Criterio diagnostico della possessione diabolica".

4 Dual and Multiple Personalities

4.1 The (Literary) Story of Dr Jekyll and Mr Hyde

The famous novel *The Strange Case of Dr Jekyll and Mr Hyde* by Robert Louis Stevenson is very well known, not least because of the numerous (even parodic) adaptations it has been subjected to during its century and a half of existence. It tells how one and the same person experiences two separate existences, in which thoughts, affections, and dominant motivations are entirely different. The text is structured in such a way as to suggest duplicity: the writing divides it into an initial part, in which the story is told by an "omniscient narrator", and a final part that consists of first-person narratives. In turn, the final part is split between the testimony of a marginal character in the unfolding of the story, but who acts as a witness, and finally the account of his own affairs written by the protagonist, Dr Jekyll.

The novel seems to progressively reveal the unpredictable links between two people who could not appear more different from each other. Jekyll is tall, good-looking, and noble-minded. Hyde is unpleasant, short in stature, and low in instincts. From the very first pages, we learn that Hyde has been appointed universal heir by Jekyll and the reasons for such a choice appear as mysterious to his notary (the co-protagonist) as to anyone else. One thinks of blackmail or some other shady affair, when in fact the simple yet incredible explanation is that Jekyll and Hyde can be traced back to the same human being. The second, more obscure personality was born following the discovery of a particular chemical compound, capable of transforming the good doctor into his sinister *alter ego*. Hyde is nothing more than the embodiment of the crudely instinctive and unconscious world of the magnanimous doctor. It should be kept in mind that *The Strange Case of Dr Jekyll and Mr Hyde* was published in 1886, ten years before Freud first used the word "psychoanalysis".[1] The time was evidently ripe for the psychoanalytic revolution.

In Henry Jekyll's "Full Statement of the Case", the final chapter, a long passage explains what the assumptions of the transformation experiment are:

DOI: 10.4324/9781003481249-5

> With every day, and from both sides of my intelligence, the moral and the intellectual, I thus drew steadily nearer to that truth, by whose partial discovery I have been doomed to such a dreadful shipwreck: that man is not truly one, but truly two. I say two, because the state of my own knowledge does not pass beyond that point. Others will follow, others will outstrip me on the same lines; and I hazard the guess that man will be ultimately known for a mere polity of multifarious, incongruous and independent denizens.[2]

This literary intuition was destined for a paradoxical confirmation, as we shall see in this chapter. In any case, Jekyll's confession continues: "I saw that, of the two natures that contended in the field of my consciousness, even if I could rightly be said to be either, it was only because I was radically both".[3] Hence the idea arose in Jekyll of isolating the two potential personalities by making them, in some way, different individuals. When the experiment succeeds, a second personality reveals itself: "At the first breath of this new life", says Jekyll, "I knew myself to be more wicked, tenfold more wicked, sold a slave to my original evil; and the thought, in that moment, braced and delighted me like wine. I stretched out my hands, exulting in the freshness of these sensations".[4]

This personality is different, but also related to the original: "This, too, was myself".[5] However, while the two personalities retain "some of the phenomena of consciousness", apart from the fact that the death of one would have meant the death of the other, their memory is not perfectly common. In the case of a final option for either, "Jekyll would suffer smartingly in the fires of abstinence, Hyde would be not even conscious of all that he had lost".[6] Jekyll and Hyde's capacities also differ: "I have more than once observed", the protagonist notes, "that, in my second character, my faculties seemed sharpened to a point and my spirits more tensely elastic".[7] Above all, however, the two end up considering themselves as distinct also from the point of view of their respective responsibilities: "It was Hyde, after all, and Hyde alone, that was guilty. Jekyll was no worse; he woke again to his good qualities seemingly unimpaired; he would even make haste, where it was possible, to undo the evil done by Hyde. And thus his conscience slumbered".[8]

Stevenson's novel is just one of many literary incarnations of the theme of the double, known since antiquity and traceable in the Homeric poems and in Plato's *Symposium*. The theme of the double has many variations: a character splits because they lose their shadow or mirror image (which begin to live a life of their own); or they live two different, parallel lives; or they encounter a second self, which has opposite psychological characteristics. This narrative *topos* has been embodied countless times, especially since the 19th century, the century in which the existence of cases of "dual personality" began to be mentioned in reality and not only in fiction.

4.2 The Story of Félida X.

"In June 1858", Eugene Azam wrote, "I was called upon to provide care for a young commoner, Félida X., who was said to be suffering from mental alienation and who presented singular phenomena of spontaneous catalepsy, anaesthesia, hyperaesthesia. She also presented an interesting lesion [sic] of memory",[9] which he then defined as "doubling of personality or periodic amnesia".[10] Azam described himself as someone unwilling to accept the reality of alleged extraordinary phenomena naively, but also open-minded enough not to reject a priori the veracity of apparently scientifically inexplicable phenomena. After all, the limitations that psychology and physiology presented in their ability to explain the mind and brain were well known. With this attitude he prepared himself to observe the patient who would bring him fame and essentially open a long season of studies on the "subconscious", culminating in the works of Pierre Janet, one of the pioneers of modern psychotherapy.

Félida X. was born in 1843 in Bordeaux, into a family that would have been in good financial shape if her father, a merchant navy captain, had not died too early, leaving her mother in the position of having to accept menial jobs to support her children. Félida's early years were therefore difficult. At the age of 13, Félida, described as having a good intelligence, had been initiated into work as a textile worker, in which she had shown herself to be well versed. At the same time she had begun to manifest hysterical symptoms: "various nervous accidents, pulmonary haemorrhages, inexplicable on the basis of the condition of the respiratory organs".[11] At the age of 14, however, an entirely new condition had manifested itself for the first time. When she felt a strong emotion, Félida would feel a pain in her temples and remain in a state of apparent drowsiness for about ten minutes. After this time, she would enter a state that Azam called *condition seconde* ("condition two") for an hour or two, only to return to her previous drowsiness and finally to her normal state. The phenomenon, initially sporadic, ended up occurring once a day at least and it was at this point, in 1858, that the parents requested Azam's intervention as an alienist. According to Azam, in condition two:

> [Félida] raises her head and, opening her eyes, greets the people around her with a smile, as if they had just arrived; her physiognomy, which before had appeared sad and silent, lights up and becomes cheerful; her speech is brief and she continues the needlework she had begun in her previous state; she gets up and her walk is agile, while she barely notices the thousands of pains that a few minutes before were making her suffer; she devotes herself to daily activities, she goes around the city, she pays visits [...] her way of moving and her cheerfulness are those of a girl of her age [...]. But her character has completely changed: from sad she has become cheerful and her vivacity borders on turbulence.[12]

All her perceptive and intellectual faculties seem to be more developed. In appearance, there are no symptoms of a psychotic character: no delirium, no hallucinations, no fixed ideas. In her second condition, Félida does not lose the memory of what she had experienced, done, thought in her normal, ordinary state. She also recovers the memory of her previous experiences in the second condition, which, conversely, she seems to lose when she re-enters the first. In this Félida, as can be seen, recalls the way Stevenson imagined the relationship between Hyde's memory and Jekyll's. Félida re-enters into the first condition after three to four hours. She goes again through a phase of apparent sleep and returns to the sad and aching girl she was before. All this, Azam reports, occurs once a day, at the time he is called in for consultation. Rarely, Félida also finds herself in a third condition (which Azam, however, considers to be in essence a specific modification of the second), which lasts very little and during which she seems to manifest panic attacks – she simply says: "I'm afraid! I'm afraid!"

The psychological experience of Félida's condition two is, according to Azam, so inaccessible to the former that it leads to truly paradoxical consequences. Félida becomes pregnant during an experience of condition two and willingly accepts the idea of having a child, whereas when she returns to her original condition, she does not seem to understand the changes that progressively affect her body and worries about the possibility of suffering from a disease that makes her gain weight.

Azam also makes observations on Félida using hypnosis, thanks to which he seems to be able to take his patient from one condition to another with relative ease. However, while the idea of a possible curative effect of hypnosis prompted him, in addition to scientific curiosity, this intention was not followed by any results. Between 1859 and 1876 Azam lost track of Félida. In the meantime, she married the young man who had made her pregnant and became pregnant ten more times, although only two children survived.

According to her husband's testimony to Azam, Félida went through periods in which the two conditions alternated in different ways. If initially the second condition occupied a tenth of her life, it gradually came to equal the first condition in duration, until it almost completely substituted it. The exceptional state practically supplanted the other and became the norm. Azam was prompted to get back in touch with Félida because cases similar to this were now being described by many other authors and he himself wanted to enrich his previous material for publication. He noticed how distressing the brief periods of the first condition, in which the woman continued to lose her memory of what was happening to her in the other.

Azam, however, noted that those who have dealt with similar phenomena had often described complete splits of the personality, i.e. situations in which two different persons seemed to alternate within the same body, to the point of sometimes even taking different names. Félida's situation appeared different, and Azam finally defined it as "periodic amnesia and apparent doubling of life".[13] Nevertheless, Félida's case goes down in history as the prototype of double personality cases. Such is in fact considered especially under the impetus of Pierre Janet, who refers to it in these terms in a seminal book, *Psychological Automatism.*[14]

4.3 Double Personality

In order to introduce the theme of double personality, we resorted to a "double" narrative introduction. In Stevenson's story, it is Jekyll who decides on his own to summon Hyde and succeeds in doing so by resorting to a kind of magic potion which, in the century of the scientific revolution in biology and medicine, is identified with an unknown chemical compound, synthesised in a laboratory. Azam describes Félida as being characterised by two different "conditions", not by two different identities (plus a third one, which, however, seems to be strongly linked to the second). In fact, even between Jekyll and Hyde, there is no total separation. In other cases, however, one has distinct personalities that know about each other, but also personalities that are completely unaware of each other. In other words, in the same person, two identities would coexist that take turns taking control of the body.

Fantasies about the dual nature of human personality, as mentioned above, have ancient roots. After all, ethical dilemmas have often been occasionally interpreted as the presence of two souls in the same man since ancient Greek times, if not even earlier.[15] On the other hand, descriptions of real (or at least purportedly real) cases of double personality began to be published, albeit very sporadically, from the end of the 18th century in Europe and the United States. Until the mid-19th century, however, they accounted for just a few rare cases. A peak in observations occurred in the late 19th and early 20th century, with an epicentre in France. Thereafter, the phenomenon practically disappeared from the radar of clinical observation to resurge, although modified, in the United States at the end of the 20th century. Europe was apparently only affected by it as a consequence. From the two (sporadically three or four) personalities of the first wave, in fact, a much more variable number (even dozens) appeared, which explains why the expression "multiple personality" began to be used instead of "double personality".

According to Ellenberger,[16] the observation of the first cases of double personality was only possible when the idea of demonic possession slowly began to wane.[17] Whether or not there is a historical connection between the decline in the number of possessed persons and the appearance of double personality, the first known historical example of such a pathology comes not long after the controversy between the exorcist Gassner and the "magnetist" Mesmer, and dates from the time of the outbreak of the French Revolution. In 1791, a German neurologist published the case of a young girl who, impressed by the manners of the young French aristocrats who had fled their homeland at the time of the storming of the Bastille, unwittingly began to take on a new personality that imitated their characteristics, even going so far as to express herself in French instead of German.

Erasmus Darwin reported that he had cured, by administering opium, a lady of high social standing and good intellectual gifts, who would indulge in thought and reverie every other day, only to resume it later, leading his acquaintances to think that she had like two separate minds. In 1815, the case of Mary Reynolds came to light. For 15 years or so she had been subject to the transition, passing, through a fainting spell and a subsequent sleep, into a second personality in which she "became restless and eccentric; she wandered off into the woods without concern for wolves and bears and once attempted to catch a rattlesnake. She was also under the spell of a brother-in-law".[18]

In some cases, the two personalities appeared independent and even mutually amnesic, to the point of taking two different names. William James studied the case of Ansel Bourne who, already presumed to have been miraculously converted, became a preacher and disappeared from his home in Rhode Island. He presented himself a few days later as Albert Brown in a small town in Pennsylvania and opened a business there. Waking up one morning, two months later, disoriented and completely unaware of how he came to be in his new home, Ansel Bourne returned to his former life with no recollection of his life as Albert Brown, except that he could recall everything under hypnosis (in this respect, his story is certainly reminiscent of that of the "mad traveller" Albert Dadas).[19] The circumstances, however, generated some suspicion: Bourne had disappeared after withdrawing a large sum of money from the bank and was apparently afflicted by the "nagging" character of his second wife.[20]

The numerous cases studied by Pierre Janet were also marked by the assumption of different names for the different personalities. The second personality could present different tastes, preferences for different people, write letters in a different style, and complain about the first personality. Even when looking at Janet's accounts, however, doubts about the authenticity of the phenomenon are legitimate. Consider the following passage from *Psychological Automatism*. The author recounts a dialogue that had taken place between himself and a patient by means of "automatic writing", i.e. a situation in which a person would move the pen without being aware of what they are actually writing.

> Having noticed, I admit with some astonishment, the secondary intelligence which was manifested by Lucie's automatic writing, one day I had the following conversation with her while her normal self was chatting with another person. 'Do you hear me?' I say to her. (She answers in writing), 'No'. 'But in order to answer, you have to hear'. 'Yes, absolutely'. 'So how do you do it?' 'I do not know'. I ask, 'Does someone have to hear me?' 'Yes'. 'Who is that?' 'Someone other than Lucie'. 'Ah! Someone else. Do you want us to give them a name?' 'No'. 'Yes, it will be more convenient'. She responded, 'Well then, Adrienne'. 42 'So, Adrienne, can you hear me?' She responded, 'Yes'. No doubt it was I who suggested that she name this personage and thus gave her a sort of

individuality, but one can see how far she had already developed in that direction spontaneously.[21]

In fact, the same story had previously been told differently: the name proposed by Janet was Blanche,[22] but upon waking up Lucie had found this name unbearable, and it was agreed to replace it with Adrienne. This is how Ian Hacking comments on the episode:

> The anecdote is somewhat naive. One can observe a great influence of 'suggestion', to borrow the sceptical comments of Hippolyte Bernheim, a doctor in Nancy and a severe critic of Parisian infatuations and enthusiasms. One might think that Pierre Janet did not 'discover' a hidden personality, but that he created it. We, sophisticated auditors, think that Adrienne (or Blanche) came into being thanks to Janet's intervention. He truly made Adrienne a reality. He moulded this personality, and the act of naming her Adrienne is essential to this moulding.[23]

"Once baptised, the unconscious personage", i.e. the secondary personality, of which the former has no awareness, "is more determined and sharper. It displays its psychological characteristics better".[24] It seems clear, then, that the "baptism" on the part of the scholar contributes a great deal to constructing the alleged "other". In any case, Janet's awareness of the possibility that he himself induced phenomena of suggestion emerges clearly in *Psychological Automatism*: the people he studies, he says, undergo his influence "like little children. They believe everything that enters their mind".[25]

Shall we say then that the idea of double personality could be an invention, that the relevant cases were iatrogenic, i.e. induced by doctors' suggestion? The answer may not be straightforward. Hacking himself, returning to the question on three occasions, provides three different answers. In a short essay from the 1980s, Hacking expresses no doubts about the belief that double personality was never a real clinical phenomenon but was created by its purported observers. In an extensive book from the following decade, written after the explosion of the multiple personality phenomenon in the United States, Hacking is more nuanced and, although evidently sceptical, prefers a phenomenological description, not without humorous tones though, to clear-cut, definitive judgement. In the course at the Collège de France, ten years later, Hacking's "constructivist" stance prompts him to assert that it is somehow useless (or irrelevant) to separate supposedly authentic clinical phenomena from those resulting from the influence of observers, because such phenomena are always and in any case the result of co-construction.

However, what is certainly not the result of invention is the idea that the human personality – no matter how one wants to define it – is anything but unique. Reconsider the literary theme of the double, which has fascinated writers and storytellers throughout the ages, but began to be used especially since the 19th century. Various narrators have imagined human beings encountering another self, in the form of a strangely physically similar person, who may be better (Poe's *William Wilson*) or worse (Stevenson's *The Master of Ballantrae*), complementary (Conrad's *The Secret Sharer*) or persecutory (Dostoevsky's *The Double*); an image that takes on a life of its own, such as the shadow (Chamisso's *Peter Schlemhil*), a portrait (Wilde's *The Portrait of Dorian Gray*), the mirror, and which can also be constructed or conjured up by the protagonist (Mary Shelley's *Frankenstein*).

One of the pioneers of psychoanalysis, Otto Rank, dedicated a book entitled *The Double: A Psychoanalytic Study* to this theme, arguing that literature had merely thematised in an imaginative way a fact that psychoanalysis had instead scientifically ascertained: the existence of the unconscious. In writers who had proposed variations on this theme, according to Rank, "the fantasy of the other self is a projection of its inner split".[26] In this sense, the split personality, instead of being experienced in one's own life, would have been projected by the writers into the paper existence of their protagonists. Regardless of the validity of Rank's thesis, the theme of the double was continually and abundantly revisited throughout the 20th century and the first decades of the new century, not only in literature but also, in films. On the contrary, the pathology of the double personality first almost completely disappeared and then reappeared on the scene, although multiplying the number of "others" besides the original "ego".

4.4 Multiple Personality

Following Ian Hacking's historical reconstruction, those who had looked in scientific publications during the early 1970s for traces of cases of double/multiple personalities referred to the previous 50 years would have been able to count only very few, at most a few dozen worldwide and always reported as mere curiosities and certainly not as prototypes of a widespread condition.[27] Nevertheless, in 1980, the definition of multiple personality disorder entered the Diagnostic and Statistical Manual of Mental Diseases and by 1982 there was already talk of an epidemic of cases, at least in the United States.

In 1986, it could be estimated that 6000 patients had already been diagnosed, and within a further five years, every US city of a certain size could count hundreds of such cases. After that, the number diagnosed would have to be estimated as a percentage of the total population, reaching a paradoxical 5%. The reason for such a fluctuation was, according to Hacking, due to a change in the clinical paradigm. At the end of the 19th century, the scene of psychopathology was occupied by hysterical manifestations, and double personality was considered to be a sort of by-product of hysteria; by declining diagnoses of hysteria and related phenomena, dual personality would similarly be forgotten as a possible diagnosis.

The late 20th century devoted special attention to child abuse, rediscovering the phenomena of personality dissociation once studied by Janet. This entailed either a greater focus on a diagnosis long overlooked – and thus the identification of cases that had simply eluded observers for a long time – or a construction or co-construction of invented cases. Hacking seems to prefer this second explanation, which he corroborates among other things with the discovery of the false memory syndrome, linked to iatrogenic suggestion, which leads to the reconstruction of abuse that never really happened. Even the passage that has occurred, from a few cases of double personality to innumerable cases of the co-presence of dozens of alternative personalities in the same sufferers, seems to Hacking a clear indication of possible cultural construction, exacerbated by the popularity of the phenomenon, as indicated among other things also by the success of MPD biographies/autobiographies. Frank Putnam himself, one of the most well-known scholars on the subject, wrote: "An elaborate mythology has grown up around alter personalities. Unfortunately, certain MPD therapists and patients have fed this mythology themselves, and thus it is not easily dispelled".[28]

Starting from the same historical data taken into account by Hacking, however, the reconstruction of what happened can be very different. In Janet's model, the neurotic condition was always linked to more or less severe forms of *dissociation* of the personality. Dissociative phenomena would in this sense constitute a continuum, from everyday forms of occasional loss of attention to the actual splitting of the personality, passing through different forms of amnesia (loss of memory), analgesia (insensitivity to pain), acts performed unconsciously (or subconsciously), fixed ideas. According to a well-known contemporary clinician:

> [Dissociative symptoms] involve intrusions, e.g., additional sensations, movements, and perceptions, up to the extremes of complete interruptions of the habitual state of consciousness through reactivations of dissociative *secondary existences*. These dissociative states display psychological and somatoform features which diverge from those characteristic of the habitual state.[29]

However, Freud's *psychoanalysis*, which in the course of the 20th century clearly won the cultural battle against Janet's *psychological medicine*, long favoured the establishment of a model in which neurosis was rather explained by the conflict of unconscious motives than by dissociation. Only recently have Janet's ideas begun to be re-evaluated, even within the field of psychoanalysis itself.[30] According to Frank Putnam, in fact:

> From our late-20th-century perspective, the disappearance of the dissociative disorders from mainstream psychology and psychiatry at the beginning of the century appears to have been driven by concerns about

> the credibility of MPD and fears that cases were being iatrogenically produced in suggestible patients. Other influences – such as the inclusion of MPD patients under the diagnosis of schizophrenia, the rise of psychoanalytic theory with its emphasis on repression, and experiments by Messerschmidt 'disproving' the independence of dissociated processes – also contributed to a loss of interest in dissociation after the 1920s. The decline in the use of dissociative diagnoses is evidence that aggressive challenges to credibility can lead to their disuse in mainstream psychiatry.[31]

In fact, the concept of dissociation has become so widely accepted in contemporary clinical psychology that a prestigious journal is devoted solely to this topic and bears the unequivocal title *Dissociation*. The well-known *Defence Mechanisms Rating Scale* (DMRS) includes dissociation among neurotic defences (thus not among the most severe).[32]

In the meantime, however, Multiple Personality Disorder, in the editions following the third, has been absorbed into a more generic category, taking on the name Dissociative Identity Disorder (DID). In the definition offered by the DSM-5-TR, DID is marked by "disruption of identity characterized by two or more distinct personality states".[33] It is precisely the media popularity achieved by certain cases that have probably led clinicians to use more cautious language. According to the new perspective, Putnam specifies: "Alter personalities are real. They do exist—not as separate individuals, but as discrete dissociative states of consciousness. When considered from this perspective, they are not nearly so amazing to behold or so difficult to accept".[34] Actually, cases of multiple personalities with completely different names and characters have again disappeared from clinical descriptions and media reports. One might wonder, however, whether the moments of resounding affirmation of the phenomenon were due to collusion between patients and clinicians; or whether, on the contrary, distrust gradually led clinicians to consider real cases fictitious.

Notes

1 Freud, *Heredity*; *Further Remarks*.
2 Stevenson, *The Strange Case of Dr Jekyll and Mr Hyde*, 108.
3 Stevenson, *The Strange Case of Dr Jekyll and Mr Hyde*, 108.
4 Stevenson, *The Strange Case of Dr Jekyll and Mr Hyde*, 112.
5 Stevenson, *The Strange Case of Dr Jekyll and Mr Hyde*, 114.
6 Stevenson, *The Strange Case of Dr Jekyll and Mr Hyde*, 125.
7 Stevenson, *The Strange Case of Dr Jekyll and Mr Hyde*, 132.
8 Stevenson, *The Strange Case of Dr Jekyll and Mr Hyde*, 119.
9 Azam, *Hypnotisme*, 12.
10 Azam, *Hypnotisme*, 61.
11 Azam, *Hypnotisme*, 63.
12 Azam, *Hypnotisme*, 67–68.

13 Azam, *Hypnotisme*, 109.
14 Janet, *L'Automatisms Psychologique.*
15 Capizzi, *L'uomo a due anime.*
16 Ellenberger, *The Discovery of the Unconscious.*
17 Conversely, in more recent times, the concept of dual and multiple personalities has been used as a key to the explanation of possession phenomena in non-European cultures (e.g., Suryani and Jensen, *Trance and Possession in Bali*).
18 Ellenberger, *The Discovery of the Unconscious*, 128–129.
19 See chapter 5.
20 Ellenberger, *The Discovery of the Unconscious*, 135.
21 Janet, *L'automatisme psychologique*, vol. 2, 64.
22 Janet, "Les actes inconscients".
23 Hacking, *Façonner les gens*, 34–35.
24 Hacking, *Façonner les gens*, 35
25 Janet, *L'automatisme psychologique*, vol. 1, 141.
26 Rank, *The Double*, 57.
27 Hacking, *Rewriting the Soul*
28 Putnam, *Dissociation*, 90.
29 Nijenhuis, *Somatoform Dissociation*, 12; italics in the original.
30 See, e.g., Bromberg, *Standing in the Spaces*; *Awakening the Dreamer*: *The Shadow of the Tsunami.*
31 Putnam, *Dissociation*, 4–5; omitted references.
32 Perry, *Defense Mechanism Rating Scales*; Di Giuseppe and Perry, "The Hierarchy of Defence Mechanisms", 9.
33 APA, *DSM-5-TR*, 330.
34 Putnam, *Dissociation*, 90.

5 Mad Travellers

5.1 The Story of Albert

In June 1886. Albert Dadas, a gas worker in Bordeaux, while in conversation with doctor Philippe Tissié, does not seem to have a very clear idea of his identity and what has recently happened to him. "How old are you", he is asked. "Maybe 29", he replies. He was actually born in 1860, making him 26. Tissié informs him. Albert says he is happy to learn his age for sure.

The next day Tissié asks Albert the same question: "How old are you?" Albert replies that he remembers how the doctor asked him the day before, but he has absolutely no recollection of the answer. After such a beginning, not many would have hoped to get much out of such a patient, but Tissié does not lose his trust. He decides to reconstruct what Albert apparently does not remember by hypnotising him, exactly as Breuer tried to do in the same years with Anna O.

Under hypnosis Albert remembers.

Hospitalised in 1886 for amnesia following an "escape", after which he cannot say when or why he left the town where he lived, worked, and had asked a girl to marry him, Albert says he was by no means new to such an experience. In fact, in the course of his life, it happened several times that he went into a kind of *trance* and found himself in an unknown place without knowing why. Or rather, sometimes he might even know why: he had heard about a faraway and fascinating place and had thought it would be nice to get there. But then he was on his way, or already in the place he had longed for, typically having lost money and documents on the way, without having any consciousness of having decided to leave.

The story began in 1872. Twelve years old, Albert Dadas, was working as an apprentice at a gas appliance manufacturer in Bordeaux. Working as a boy was common at the time. It was less common for a 12-year-old apprentice to leave his job in his hometown and find another one a few kilometres away, without telling his parents. Completely unprecedented it seemed that the same person had not realised the change. Albert, who had disappeared without saying anything, was in fact found in La Teste by his brother. In the meantime, he had become a clerk for an umbrella-maker, alongside whom he

DOI: 10.4324/9781003481249-6

had wandered around the province. "What are you doing in La Teste?" his brother asked him, patting him on the back. Albert had had something of an awakening. He did not know why he was there.

It is only the first in a series of episodes. He hears mention of a nearby city in which his father is to receive some sort of inheritance and finds himself there a few days later with no memory of how he got there. He hears mention of Paris and is found sleeping on a park bench in the capital.

His story goes on like this, with increasingly frequent outward journeys, longer and longer, and increasingly uncomfortable return journeys, complicated by the fact that in the meantime Albert Dadas has again lost his papers and spent the money he had in his pocket (sometimes even the money he had been entrusted with for an errand). But Albert adapts and always finds a good soul who gives him a few francs and some piecework to make ends meet. He learns to live with running away and acquires extraordinary training in the ability to move on foot. Some of his fellow adventurers die of exhaustion, but not him.

The journeys, as time goes by, become increasingly longer and more and more daring. He hears about Marseilles and finds himself in Marseilles. In Marseilles, he hears about Africa and leaves for Africa. At this point Albert acquires another important notion for his survival: abroad there is always a French consul willing to provide new documents and generally some money for the return journey.

Twice he joins the military and twice he defects. He crosses the border permanently and the journeys become even more complicated. His new base, instead of his hometown, becomes Vienna, where a Frenchman re-employs him as a worker in a gas company. Several times he also leaves Vienna, and several times he returns there to be reemployed. Apparently, when he works Albert is appreciated for his commitment to what he is asked to do.

In the end, however, Albert does not have the courage to return to Vienna after yet another escape. He leaves for the north. The advice he receives is not always the right one: "Go to that castle and they will feed you!" they tell him. He goes and almost gets mauled by a dog. "Go to Moscow, which is full of French people and they will certainly help you!" they tell him. And he goes to Moscow and is arrested. Luckily for him, the Russians simply expel him from the country, transporting him to the Turkish border. There he finds himself, without knowing how, in Constantinople. He then begins yet another long journey back across Europe, which finally brings him, amidst various travails, to Bordeaux. Where Albert, for a while, seems to play the role of the prodigal son. He goes back to work hard in a gas company, falls in love with a girl, and asks her to marry him. The wedding is arranged but – who would believe it! – Albert disappears again without realising what he is up to.

Finally admitted to a hospital, he meets Philippe Tissié, who tells his story. Tissié, however, does not just listen to Albert Dadas but seeks information from his family, the employers where Albert says he was employed, and the military departments where he says he enlisted. The feedback he receives seems to confirm what Albert remembers under hypnosis. Paradoxically, in fact, under hypnosis Albert recalls extremely minute details, compared to the conscious condition of a person who does not even know his own age. In fact, Albert reports every country from which he passed, every sum he was bestowed or paid for his work, every *corvée* he performed in exchange for passage or hospitality.

Tissié observes Albert at length and uses his case as the subject of his doctoral thesis, which became a book entitled *The Mad Travellers.*[1]

Albert is the first "mad traveller".

5.2 The Brief History of Mad Travellers

The subject of mad travelling has been specifically studied by Jean-Claude Beaune and Ian Hacking.[2] The Canadian epistemologist, in particular, considered *dromomania*,[3] *poriomania*,[4] or *ambulatory automatism*[5] as the typical example of "transient mental illness", which Hacking defines as "an illness that appears at a time, in a place, and later fades away".[6] Albert is indeed the first in a short but intense sequence of similar cases. As Hacking writes, it was Albert who initiated "an epidemic of fugues, or better, it was Tissié" who initiated "an epidemic of diagnoses of fugues".[7] Such a diagnostic epidemic, however, would probably not have occurred without the specific interest of Charcot, who dealt with the subject several times.[8]

In fact, as German Berrios points out, cases qualifying as escapes are described in France even before the meeting between Albert Dadas and Philippe Tissié:

> Descriptions of behaviours similar to ' fugues' can be found at least since 1851, when Aubanel reported the case of a patient with neurosyphilis who used to escape in a bewildered state. [...] The term 'fugue' seems to have been first used by Lasègue in 1868 to refer to the symptoms of an alcoholic subject during a dreamy, hallucinatory state. The first important monograph on the topic is that by Achilles Foville who described a series of 13 subjects [...] with a tendency to wandering away from home.[9]

The (diagnostic) epidemic of mad travellers, in any case, originated in Bordeaux, developed for a few decades mainly in the same area, but then also saw cases in the rest of France and, sporadically, beyond the Alps and the Rhine. In Prussian territory, one wonders why no one has described cases of mad travellers, and here at last come timely accounts in the German-speaking world.[10] Further east, finally, mad travellers are spoken of in Russia,[11] a country whose culture was very attentive to the French world between the 19th and early 20th century.

The profile of the mad traveller seems to have a fairly precise location not only from a historical-geographical point of view but also from a social one:

> The fugueur was no average man on the road. He was sober, clean, respectable, a member of the working poor, by no means permanently destitute. An artisan, a delivery man, a clerk, a small shopkeeper, not to be confused with the broad mass of tramps and vagrants whom the French population in the 1880s came increasingly to see as a fundamental social problem. The fugueur was not from the middle classes. But he was urban or had a trade. There are almost no reports of peasant or farmer fugueurs.[12]

The context in which the figure of the mad traveller arises has specific characteristics that are worthy of attention. Until recently before Albert's case, the idea of journeying was mainly linked to three possible circumstances: a pilgrimage to holy places (e.g. to Rome, on the occasion of the Jubilee, to receive an indulgence); a transfer linked to work or specific reasons connected to the activity of travelling salesmen; and the pleasure and self-education of very wealthy people (Montaigne, Goethe, Byron, Stendhal kept travel diaries). Some innovations, however, made more popular tourism possible. Firstly, the concept previously unknown to the masses of "free time" from work emerged. It was in France that paid holidays, i.e. a short period of the year in which it is possible to rest, came into being. Secondly, someone, such as Thomas Cook, came up with the possibility of offering relatively inexpensive travel for pleasure trips for groups of people. Thirdly, the invention of the velocipede, later perfected into the bicycle, made it possible to move with relatively little one-off cost and at moderate speed from one city to another. Singularly, the arrival of the first competitive bicycle race destined to become a "classic" (the Paris-Bordeaux, in fact) is located in Bordeaux.

There is, however, a fourth remarkable circumstance, which favours the location of the mad traveller in France. It is the identification and then the sanction of the status of vagrant. As early as 1790, shortly after the start of the Revolutionary period, it was established that beggars were to be traced back to their communes of origin, but it was not until 1810 that the French penal code recognised the figure of the "vagabond" as a person to be identified with a *marque*. And only in 1818, the law specified the conditions under which vagrancy was to be identified as a crime, with its own criminal intention and its corresponding act of commission. In this sense, the vagrant was a person to be punished by arrest if they had no trade, no home, no means of subsistence. The phenomenon of vagrancy seems to have peaked around 1890, when tens of thousands were arrested on this charge in France and then declined sharply at the beginning of the 20th century.[13] If one parallels these dates with the rise and fall of the phenomenon of ambulatory automatism, one is led to think, firstly, that the spread of collective attention to vagrancy makes it easier for a person to be noticed moving from one place to another.

Secondly, it is evident that one possible interpretation of the occurrence of the supposed symptoms is an attempt to avoid the charge of vagrancy and the risk of jail. This opens up a question, to which it is impossible to give an objective answer: how much do mad travellers simulate their condition?

That the symptoms of the *fugueurs* are thus, to some extent, a reflection of the times and customs seems quite evident. However, another aspect of the subject of the mad travellers is worthy of attention. Somehow the ambulatory automatism quickly became a sort of second-rate transitory mental illness. Doctors and psychiatrists were not satisfied with the classification (not "scientific enough"?) and tried to place fugueurs within pre-existing nosographic categories. Some considered the symptoms to be related to epilepsy. Others preferred to trace them back to a mental illness that is itself considered transient in Hacking's terms: conversion hysteria.

It is worth opening a digression at this point. While epilepsy can certainly not be considered a transitory disease, the hypothesis of an epileptic focus reflected the beliefs of a broad school of French psychiatry at the time. The origin of this school was Antoine Laurent Jessé Bayle's *Treatise on the Diseases of the Brain and its Membranes*,[14] which proposed that all mental illnesses could be traced back to specific lesions or inflammations of the brain. Bayle's theses were contested by Esquirol and his pupils[15] and this dualism spanned the entire 19th century. The opposition was to be followed up in the dualism between "functionalists" and "localizationists" in neurology. Even those who were convinced of the inseparable link between mind and brain, in fact, debated whether every aspect of the mind's activity was carried out by a precise area of the brain (localisation of function) or instead by a system of neuronal connections without a unique and identifiable location. For example, Freud's book on aphasia was an expression of such a debate. Freud, a functionalist, argued against the localisationists precisely in an area where they seemed to have achieved their first successes.[16]

One might think that a further usable diagnostic category might have been that of double personality (itself a "transient mental illness"). Tissié met Eugène Azam at one point, who had in turn described the case of Félida X, the archetype of double personality cases. Azam, however, comparing Albert's case with Félida's, ruled out the possibility of the same diagnosis:

> In summary, Albert X was affected by a general neurosis of the order of hysteria, which, although rare in men, has nevertheless been observed several times [...]. Albert X's amnesia is not comparable to that of Félida. It is more complete, more profound; Albert loses, in fact, the recollection of everything he had learned and of so-called general ideas [...]. Therefore, he never had the connotations of a doubling of personality.[17]

Almost all the cases of double personality observed in France were of women. One could jokingly point out that if Albert had been diagnosed as a double personality, male cases would have been harder to find because they were busy wandering from one city to another. Nevertheless, since the hysteria cases were also fundamentally female, *fugueurs* as hysterics might have filled another vacant box.

However, as mentioned above, while the possibility of tracing the mad travellers' syndrome back to hysteria was hypothesised, epilepsy was also considered:

> The two great but mysterious mental pathologies of the day were hysteria and epilepsy. Bordeaux said that fugue was a hysterical condition. Paris said that it was latent epilepsy. Peacemakers said that some fugues are hysterical while others are epileptic. This issue, once burning, has been extinguished to the point where we find it hard to make sense of. Yet it was part of the environment that enabled fugue diagnoses to thrive.[18]

Someone also proposed that some forms of ambulatory automatism could be epileptic, others hysterical, and finally others of toxic origin.[19] Charcot spoke of possible "hysteron-epilepsy", i.e. a disease that synthesised the other two. The debate lost force and significance when the observed cases of insane travellers declined, as quickly as they had peaked.

5.3 Epilogue: Other Times, Other Places, Other Escapes

It was suggested in the 1980s that the concept of escape, as a symptomatic behaviour involving actual movement through space, evolved through three different epochs: the first is the one we have been considering and basically coincides with the epidemic of mad travellers, which ends in the early 1910s. The second, which lasts until the Second World War, characterises escapism as a psychomotor disorder. The last phase, which would last until the 1980s, conceives escaping as a consequence of multiple possible factors.[20]

The history of this symptom, however, takes a sharp turn with the DSM-III, but especially with the DSM-IV. Both manuals identify a syndrome characterised by "sudden, unexpected travel away from home or one's customary place of daily activities". Whereas the former identifies "psychogenic fugue" as the possible symptom of loss of identity, the latter changes the name of the syndrome to "dissociative fugue" and assumes that "confusion about personal identity or even the assumption of a new identity" would be the predominant symptom and that this requirement is fundamental to making the diagnosis.[21] The "assumption of a new (partial or complete) identity" also seems possible.[22] Dissociative fugue is considered by the DSM-IV as a possible aspect of Dissociative Identity Disorder and is generally associated with traumatic events, but it is possible that it is coexistent with "depression, dysphoria, depression, shame, guilt, psychological stress, conflict, suicidal and aggressive impulses".[23]

Meanwhile, a review article reported that a Canadian study, conducted on a *non-clinical* sample of more than a thousand people, found symptoms of dissociative amnesia in 10% of the sample, while almost 1% of the sample met the criteria for dissociative fugue.[24] The article suggested caution in considering this study and pointed out the need to replicate it, before coming to premature conclusions. The study, however, remained seemingly isolated: did it record a new small epidemic of fugueurs or was it simply poorly conducted? This too is a question that has no certain answer.

The *Text Revision* version of the DSM-IV confirms what was contained in the previous edition, while the picture changes again with the DSM-5, which declassifies "Dissociative fugue" to a possible symptom of "Dissociative amnesia".[25] One then has "Dissociative amnesia with dissociative fugue", defined as follows: "Apparently purposeful travel or bewildered wandering that is associated with amnesia for identity or for other important autobiographical information".[26]

The DSM-5 and DSM-5-TR also lose track of the section on dissociative fugue devoted to "culture-related characteristics", where we find these observations:

> Individuals with various culturally defined 'running' syndromes (e.g., *pibloktoq* among native peoples of the Arctic, *grisi siknis* among the Miskito of Honduras and Nicaragua, Navajo 'frenzy' witchcraft, and some forms of *amok* in Western Pacific cultures) may have symptoms that meet diagnostic criteria for Dissociative Fugue. These are conditions characterized by a sudden onset of a high level of activity, a trancelike state, potentially dangerous behavior in the form of running or fleeing, and ensuing exhaustion, sleep, and amnesia for the episode.[27]

It will be interesting to note, at this point, that the Navajo's "frenetic magic" was in another context indicated as a possible result of epilepsy or hysteria;[28] that the Alaskan Inuit's term "pibloqtoq" can be translated as "arctic hysteria" but has nothing to do with the pathology of the same name that this book will deal with and the doubt has been raised that its identification was fabricated in an artificial way by the relations between anthropologists and Inuit[29]; that "grisi siknis" implies a form of demonic possession.[30]

The DSM-IV also highlighted the hypothesis that forms of wandering may be associated with manic episodes, i.e. periods (at least four days) of exaggeratedly elevated mood, often characterised by hyperactivity; and also with schizophrenia, as a result of loss of contact with reality.

Indeed, one can also speak of "escape from reality" in a sense other than physical escape. It was Freud who first spoke of a possible "escape into illness" as a response to an unsatisfactory or fearful reality (and conversely of an "escape into recovery", understood as the – temporary – abandonment of symptoms in order to avoid facing one's own conflicts in psychotherapy).[31] Moreover, as we shall see, one of the most radical escapes from the world can be linked to a situation of extreme and voluntary restriction of one's space of movement.[32]

Notes

1 Tissié, *Les aliénés voyageurs.*
2 Beaune, *Le vagabond et la machine*; Hacking, *Mad Travellers.*
3 Régis, *Dromomania.*
4 Donath, "Poriomanie"; Donath, "Weitere Beiträge zur Poriomanie".
5 Alcindor and Maurat, "Un cas d'hystérie".
6 Hacking, *Mad Travellers*, 1.
7 Hacking, *Mad Travellers*, 26.
8 Charcot, *Leçons du mardi* voll. 1–2; Charcot, "Ambulatory Automatism"; Charcot, "Accès d'automatisme ambulatoire"; see also Beaune, *Le vagabond et la machine*; Goetz, "Charcot at the Salpêtrière".
9 Berrios, *History of the Mental Symptoms*, 221.
10 Burgl, "Eine Reise in die Schweiz"; Donath, "Poriomanie"; Donath, "Weitere Beiträge zur Poriomanie"; see also Hacking, *Mad Travellers*, 43.
11 Berger, "Sluchai Ambulatornogo Automatisma"; Beliaev, "Kazuistike pathologischeskikh bluzhdanii".
12 Hacking, *Mad Travellers*, 27.
13 Beaune, *Le vagabond et la machine.*
14 Bayle, *Traité des maladies du cerveau.*
15 Postel and Quétel, *Nouvelle histoire de la psychiatrie*; Pichot, *Un Siècle de psychiatrie.*
16 Freud, *Zur Auffassung der Aphasien.*
17 Azam, *Hypnotisme*, 227–228.
18 Hacking, *Mad Travellers*, 32.
19 Courtney, "The Various Forms of Ambulatory Automatism".
20 Behr, Croq, and Vauterin, "Sémiologie des conduites de fugues".
21 APA, *DSM-IV*, 481.
22 APA, *DSM-IV*, 532.
23 APA, *DSM-IV*, 530.
24 Loewenstein, "Psychogenic Amnesia and Fugue".
25 APA, *DSM-IV-TR.*
26 APA, *DSM-5*, 298; *DSM-5-TR*, 337.
27 APA, *DSM-IV-TR*, 482.
28 Levy, Neutra, and Parker, "Life Careers of Navajo Epileptics".
29 Dick, "Pibloktoq".
30 Dennis, "Grisi Siknis".
31 Freud, *Hysterical Attacks.*
32 See Chapter 9.

6 Sluggish Schizophrenia

6.1 Mikhail

We are in the 1980s, the last years of the Iron Curtain. A familiar face appears on Soviet television. Mikhail begins to talk about the shortcomings of the communist regime, the economic and food supply problems, the need for greater clarity in the management of power, and the opportunity offered for a change that would finally lead Great Mother Russia towards real progress. Two slogan-words are launched by Mikhail: *perestroika*, meaning "restructuring" (economic as well as political), and *glasnost*, meaning "transparency" (i.e. freedom of information).

Several Russian psychiatrists stand stunned in front of the TV. By the standard of the Soviet gerontocracy, full of over 70-year-olds, Mikhail, at 54, is a "young man". This alone casts him in a singular light, compared to the usual party speakers. As much as he emphasises at every turn that the necessary reforms must be carried out "in the spirit of Lenin", his words are alarming. Mikhail, according to the diagnostic categories Soviet psychiatrists have learned to apply, is certainly ill. They know that a certain specific psychiatric disorder, which they have learnt to recognise from the manuals of the legendary Professor Andrey Snezhnevsky, often begins like this. A person is convinced that there is something hidden to be revealed that only he and a few others understand and which the Communist Party is hiding; that there is something to change and reform; that Communist society is flawed (perhaps Western countries are better!). The word *glasnost* is bound to make anyone jump off their chair, since it has already been invoked by the writer Aleksandr Solzhenitsyn in his open letter to the Congress of the Union of Soviet Writers in 1967, before being expelled from the USSR.[1] The symptoms are clear and point to the typical "delusions of reformism". There can be no doubt: Mikhail suffers from sluggish schizophrenia! He must be reported immediately! He must be interned before he can cause harm to himself and others![2]

Fortunately for him, as the reader will have realised, Mikhail's surname is Gorbachev and no one has the courage to touch him, for the time being, since when he appears on television and addresses the people, including

DOI: 10.4324/9781003481249-7

psychiatrists, he is already the secretary of the Communist Party of the Soviet Union. If he is deposed from office within a few years of coming to power, it will be for reasons other than his mental health. Paradoxically, however, Gorbachev would have survived the coup attempt aimed at communist restoration unscathed. On the contrary, his manoeuvre to compromise with his enemies would be dismantled by Boris Yeltsin, who would go down in history as the "kamikaze of perestroika". The very man who had led the world out of the Cold War was in fact deposed on the charge of not being a radical enough reformer.

6.2 The Diagnosis of Schizophrenia

In order to understand the story of the psychiatrists who thought they could diagnose Gorbachev as mentally ill, a long historical-theoretical journey would be necessary, which could clarify firstly the concept of schizophrenia and how it arose; then how this concept evolved in pre-Soviet and Soviet Russia; and finally, what specific meaning the subcategory of "sluggish schizophrenia" has and what role it played in the relationship between psychiatry and the regime. Such a path can only be outlined here.

Today's conception of schizophrenia and the spectrum of psychotic disorders envisages the presence of three orders of symptoms: "positive" symptoms (i.e. characterised by the *presence* of unusual conducts), "negative" symptoms (*absence* of usual conducts) and disturbances in interpersonal relations (direct and indirect result of the pervasiveness of the other symptoms). The positive symptoms can in turn be divided into three categories: delusions, hallucinations and disorganised speech. Following the DSM, delusions are "fixed beliefs that are not amenable to change in light of conflicting evidence";[3] and hallucinations are "a perception-like experiences that occur without external stimulus. They are vivid and clear, with the full force and impact of normal perceptions, and not under voluntary control".[4] Disorganised speech is a mode of expression that is so problematic that it makes communication problematic. Negative symptoms, in summary, "include restricted affect, poverty of thought, apathy and anhedonia [*inability to feel and remember feeling pleasure*]".[5] Direct core manifestations of disturbed personal relationships are: "withdrawal, inappropriate expression of aggression and sexuality, lack of awareness of others' needs, excessive demands, and inability to have meaningful contact with other people".[6] Conversely, on an indirect level, people with such a complex relationship with reality tend to be avoided.

The specific diagnosis of schizophrenia or another form of psychosis depends on the duration and severity of the symptoms and the degree to which the patient's ability to work, study, and interact socially with others is impaired. This rather unambiguous nosographic description has been established for several years now, but it would naturally be anti-historical to use it as the sole parameter of comparison for the singular construct of schizophrenia that was developed by Soviet psychiatrists. It will therefore be appropriate to trace its origin.

The very concept of schizophrenia in fact arose a few years before the October Revolution, thanks to the Burghölzli school in Zurich, led by Eugen Bleuler, whose "lieutenant" was Carl Gustav Jung. Previously the most severe and persistent forms of madness were classified under the common label of *dementia praecox*, i.e. "premature dementia" or "precocious madness", a term that had been coined in France by Morel (*démence précoce*), but had found a fairly agreed upon definition since the fifth and especially the sixth edition of Emil Kraepelin's handbook of psychiatry.[7] Before Kraepelin, there was a tendency to categorise different forms of madness on the basis of different symptomatic descriptions. Kraepelin, on the other hand, suggested bringing them all under two basic categories, based on their deep structure and course: manic-depressive psychosis and, indeed, *dementia praecox*. In the first case, the symptoms began in adulthood, had a circular course, and did not permanently impair the patient's ability to think; in the second case, the onset was in childhood, and the symptoms progressively worsened until they led the patient to dementia.

Kraepelin's belief was in fact that early dementia could be defined as those who suffered from a deterioration of the brain that presented itself before old age. Early dementia had to be the result of a visible organic lesion and as such could only be diagnosed with certainty after the death of the sufferer through autopsy. By definition, early dementia was to be considered incurable. If a patient recovered after being considered to have dementia praecox, from Kraepelin's perspective, the diagnosis must necessarily have been wrong. The Zurich school opposed this picture. Jung began to consider the possibility that, like neurotic symptoms for Freud, psychotic symptoms could also have a psychological and symbolic meaning. They were therefore not the result of a mere physiological problem.[8] Jung, for example, had been struck by the hand gestures of an old woman who had been hospitalised for decades, which, far from being meaningless, reproduced – he discovered – the movements of the shoemaker sewing the upper of a shoe (her late husband was indeed a shoemaker). Neither Jung nor anyone else, however, ever questioned that psychosis implied a complete detachment from reality. Bleuler coined the term *schizophrenia* (from the Greek verb "skizō", i.e. to cut, to split), which emphasised the experiential dimension of the phenomenon, i.e. the splitting, precisely, of the different psychic functions, coinciding with a splitting of the patient's personality from the real world. Here is the definition offered by Bleuler:

> By the term 'dementia praecox' or 'schizophrenia' we designate a group of psychoses whose course is at times chronic, at times marked by intermittent attacks, and which can stop or retrograde at any stage, but does not permit a full *restitutio ad integrum*. The disease is characterised by a specific type of alteration of thinking, feeling and relationship to the

> external world which appears nowhere else in this particular fashion. In every case we are confronted with a more or less clear-cut splitting of the psychic function. If the disease is marked, the personality loses its unity; at different times different psychic complexes seem to represent the personality [...] Often ideas are only partially worked out, and fragments of ideas are connected in an illogical way to constitute a new idea. Concepts lose their completeness, seem to dispense with one or more of their essential components; indeed, in many cases they are only represented by a few truncated notions.[9]

Even in its original formulation, therefore, schizophrenia is defined as a loss of psychological integrity and the capacity for coherent interaction. However, it should be noted that Bleuler's consideration lent itself to being distorted and used as a precedent for the all-Soviet idea of sluggish schizophrenia:

> As a psychic process, the disease generally, if not always, begins surreptitiously. To start with, it remains latent until an acute pathological thrust produces prominent symptoms, or until a psychic shock intensifies the secondary symptoms. Often, we find a lengthy, latent period between the traumatic experience and the acute onset of the disease because the former is first subjected to elaboration.[10]

Indeed, Snezhnevsky's followers pointed to Bleuler as an illustrious Western precedent of their singular theories on "sluggishness".[11] This indication, however, was based on the circumstance that Bleuler's text, known in the Tsarist empire as early as 1912, was enormously influential on Russian psychiatrists before the October Revolution and in the 1920s and 1930s constituted an indispensable point of reference in Soviet psychiatric culture along with that of Kraepelin.[12]

6.3 Madness and Politics in Russia before Stalinism

That a regime could question the mental health of a dissident and hospitalise him is not a circumstance that occurred only in the Soviet Union (or more generally beyond the Iron Curtain during the Cold War). What is certainly peculiar to that regime, however, is (a) the systematic nature and continuity over time with which the tactic was used (hence the number of people involved and to some extent the consequent financial effort); (b) the conviction with which psychiatric diagnostic categories were applied by professionals.

With respect to point (a), it suffices to recall that in 1981 the Russian psychiatrist Anatoly Koryagin had the courage to report in the *Lancet* that the Soviet regime had opened at least 16 institutions specifically dedicated to the treatment of patients suffering from "political delusions" (i.e. opponents of the regime). Institutions to which the detention of thousands of people was entrusted.[13] Koryagin, of course, was immediately arrested and sentenced to a long prison term for anti-Soviet propaganda. Point (b) was illustrated in the reactions of some psychiatrists to Gorbachev's remarks. The first generation of mental health professionals had supposedly chosen to live with the regime or to actively collaborate for career purposes. Subsequent generations had fed on the falsifications of their masters, acquiring them as scientific truths. For many of them, certainly, the concept of sluggish schizophrenia and its applicability to those who developed "reformist delusions" were simply part of an established body of knowledge.

It can be argued that the history of pre-revolutionary and immediately post-revolutionary psychiatry somehow prepared the ground for the applicability of such a peculiar diagnosis of schizophrenia to be not only possible but logically consistent with already existing ideas. On the one hand, it may be recalled, as a historical curiosity, that the use of interning people who rebelled against the system under the pretext of a psychiatric diagnosis was by no means unknown in Tsarist Russia.[14] On the other hand, considering the diagnostic categories from beyond the Iron Curtain as a mere invention suggested by the KGB[15] constitutes a simplification, also because there is no lack of evidence of a sincere effort on the part of psychiatry in communist Europe to work with great commitment for the mental health of patients.[16]

From the very beginning, Soviet psychiatrists positioned themselves as a category well-disposed to collaborate with the regime. However, the impetus for such a willingness to collaborate was rooted in the idea that social conditions could in themselves be the source of serious mental problems for the general population.[17] The idea that work in a non-socialist society constituted a source of alienation was one of the pillars of Marx's political analysis.[18] Conversely, the therapeutic hypothesis of *ergotherapy* (occupational therapy), i.e. work (not alienated, of course) as a possible curb to psychosis certainly found fertile ground in the USSR. The now-established idea that schizophrenia could by definition have an early onset and develop with progressive worsening over time led to large-scale screening of the population: perhaps an overt condition could be prevented by occupational therapy and changing the environment of the potential sufferer.[19] Extensive research in the 1920s yielded worrying results. An enormously high number of people appeared to present or had presented psychotic symptoms such as hallucinations.[20] This led to the hypothesis that milder forms of schizophrenia existed and/or had a slower course than classical schizophrenia.

In the transition between the 1920s and the 1930s, Soviet psychological and psychiatric culture went through a period of profound change, reflecting the transition between the immediately post-revolutionary, Leninist period and the subsequent, Stalinist era. However much Lenin was still a dictator and adopted an iron fist against political opposition, some faint flames of cultural independence could also burn in the Soviet Union. On the contrary, under Stalin, the plenipotentiary minister for culture Zhdanov promoted forms of Marxist cultural orthodoxy in every field that excluded any deviation or acceptance of "Western" and "counter-revolutionary" influences.

In the field of psychiatry, this resulted in the need to interpret every observable phenomenon in the light of the concept of dialectical materialism, as suggested by the sort of manifesto that was "The Problems of Psychology in the Works of Karl Marx", by S. L. Rubinstein, published in 1934 in *Soviet Psychology*.[21] Dialectical materialism was in essence an evolution of Marx's historical materialism, which interpreted the evolution of history on the basis of the interaction (dialectic) between economic forces. This view, according to Engels and especially Lenin, could extend to nature itself, whose evolution could be interpreted in the light of the interaction of material forces. The dialectic between atoms would have produced the complex molecules. The dialectic between molecules would have generated life, and so on. In psychology and psychiatry, this meant interpreting mental phenomena solely from physiological phenomena. This implied, for example, the condemnation of psychoanalysis and all forms of phenomenological psychiatry, seen as bourgeois and decadent conceptions. The young Aleksandr Luria, for example, was an enthusiast of psychoanalysis but was induced to abandon it in order to continue his career as a scientist. Such a choice actually paid off for him, as Luria was later recognised even in the West as the founder of contemporary neuropsychology. However, this did not prevent the Communist regime from always viewing him with suspicion because he was never fully aligned with the Party's positions.

In order to avoid the purge, all psychiatrists resorted to using Ivan Pavlov's behaviourism as a reference point. The latter, although not a sympathiser of Marxism nor of the revolution, nevertheless became an indispensable point of reference for the psychiatric culture of his country and even received personal support for his research from Lenin.[22] Pavlov had introduced with his famous experiments on dogs the concept of conditioning, whereby certain behaviour, once learnt, can also manifest themselves outside the original context.

As is well known, Pavlov's dogs were measured for the amount of saliva produced after hearing the sound of a bell, which the dogs initially heard a short distance after being fed and later without being presented with food. The result was the same, showing that the dogs "salivated" at the mere perception of the *conditioned stimulus*, i.e. the perceptual stimulus they had learned to associate with the presence of food. Using behaviourism and genetic predisposition as key ideas, Soviet psychiatrists began to formulate theories that could disregard the very existence of mental processes to explain psychopathological phenomena. These principles, together with the possible "sluggishness" in the manifestation of psychosis, would open the field to dramatic consequences. During the 1930s, in fact, those ideas matured that would later allow opponents of the regime to be diagnosed as schizophrenic in a manner perfectly consistent with a doctrine: to the extent that a psychiatrist trained in the Soviet environment of that period could have made such a diagnosis *in good faith*, i.e. without the direct intention of reducing themselves to an instrument of repression in the hands of the regime.

A research group under Pyotr Gannushkin began to raise the possibility that apparently mild disorders, but characterised by apathy and introversion, masked schizophrenia.[23] One of them, Oleg Kerbikov, described in 1933 a "schizophrenia without schizophrenic symptoms", characterised by headaches, laziness, memory loss, loss of the ability to work, and decline in intellectual abilities.[24] Another group, under the leadership of V. A. Giliarovsky, identified mild forms of schizophrenia marked by mood swings and particular obsessions.[25] It was the child psychiatrist Grunya Sukhareva who coined the term "sluggish schizophrenia" (also referred to as "sluggish progressive schizophrenia"), believing that she could identify two different modes of schizophrenia development: one with a more rapid and catastrophic outcome (*malignant* schizophrenia) and the other (*sluggish* schizophrenia), which during the developmental years was characterised essentially by a tendency towards isolation and a pronounced susceptibility: mainly boys with families already marked by cases of mental disorders were subjected to it.[26] The road to the idea of a genetic dimension of schizophrenia was paved. Sukhareva also proposed classifying as *mixed* any manifestation of schizophrenia that was characterised by aspects of either form.

Dmitry Melekhov extended Sukhareva's ideas to adults.[27] It was finally Snezhnevsky, as mentioned above, who propagated a classification of schizophrenia forms that would later become the standard one in the Soviet Union. Schizophrenia was divided into *continuous*, *occasional,* and *mixed*: malignant, sluggish, and *moderate* schizophrenia became subcategories of schizophrenia with continuous manifestation. It is precisely in this classification that there was the decisive leap towards the manipulation of dissidents. The diagnosis of sluggish schizophrenia implied only the manifestation of certain insane convictions, such as "reformist delusions". For Snezhnevsky, these were devious cases, because every other aspect of thought and conduct that did not, in fact, concern political aspects, seemed absolutely normal to the observer. This was an apparent normality: precisely because of this, it made sense to isolate and keep under continuous observation not only the subject diagnosed with sluggish schizophrenia but also his or her family. Given precisely that this was a form of mental illness of genetic origin, all those who shared the same genes represented other cases of sluggish schizophrenia awaiting manifestation. Snezhnevsky gradually became a sort of undisputed leader of the Moscow School of Psychiatry, to which any possible scientific opposition, to be considered anti-Pavlovian and consequently anti-Soviet, was eliminated by the regime. Snezhnevsky paid back the regime with full cooperation. He himself, for example, diagnosed Vladimir Bukovsky as a clear case of sluggish schizophrenia.

6.4 Construction and Invention

There is an American saying that if the only tool you have is a hammer you will tend to treat any object you interact with as if it were a nail. The case of the use of the diagnosis of sluggish schizophrenia is a rather paradoxical illustration of this concept. In a way, in fact, it is as if Russian psychiatrists had been put a metaphorical hammer in their hands and told that using it on certain patients represented the only possible therapeutic solution, or at least the only possible measure for the mental hygiene of the country. Those who manifested unorthodox ideas were schizophrenic and those who were schizophrenic had to be interned and often subjected to invasive treatments of a mainly pharmacological nature. In any case, sluggish schizophrenia can be considered a diagnostic artefact, or at least the application of a concept that in reality was not completely divorced from a reconstructible context of research and thought.

It must be emphasised that the theoretical context can condition observation in many ways. Even hypotheses born in perfect good faith have historically created the premises for observations of reality distorted by erroneous assumptions. The philosophy of science has long pointed out the dangers of "the dogma of immaculate perception", which tends to ignore that everything we observe is conditioned by our system of thought. It is important to bear in mind that there are never pure data of experience. Data are always theory-laden.[28] Examples, dating back to very different historical moments, can be given to highlight this principle.

The first example concerns the definition and treatment of melancholia in the ancient Greek world. Hippocrates' conception of human physiology envisaged the existence of four humours, namely, blood, phlegm, yellow bile, and black bile. Health depended on the balance of these humours and the different characters (temperaments) depended on the relative prevalence of one of them in the body. The terms sanguine, phlegmatic, bilious, and melancholic (*mélaina kolé* means precisely black bile) are still used today, although it is hardly remembered that their origin refers to bodily fluids. Melancholia, which today we more often call depression, would have resulted from an excess of black bile. The necessary therapy would consist in eliminating this excess.

Of course, there is no such substance as black bile but, paradoxical as it may seem, the Hippocratic physicians believed that they had found a way to expel black bile from the body and could also verify that the expulsion had taken place. Probably by observing the spontaneous behaviour of certain animals such as goats, which ate hellebore leaves to purge themselves, the Hippocratic physicians noted that the resulting faeces showed an abundance of black fluid. They therefore believed that hellebore promoted the elimination of what seemed to them to be nothing more than the phantom black bile and prescribed its use to their patients, with the same result. The black liquid they observed, however, was blood subjected to intestinal digestion:

hellebore is toxic and causes copious bleeding in the stomach. The Greeks, therefore, thought they were observing a real therapeutic result (the black bile expelled from the body) and did not realise that they were instead seeing the dangerous symptom of poisoning.[29]

One might smile at such an example, thinking that only an archaic culture could introduce such primitive observation methodologies as to induce such gross errors of assessment. However, even during the 20th century, psychiatric research produced remarkable aberrations based on erroneous evaluative assumptions. On the one hand, theoretical models such as psychoanalysis and phenomenology tried to set up their attempts to treat psychosis on the basis of the patient's subjective experience. On the other hand, approaches have instead taken into account the *behaviour* of the mentally ill person, assuming that modes of acting more acceptable to the social context were the outcome to be pursued. This meant that less exaggerated and more cooperative behaviour on the part of a schizophrenic after a lobotomy was considered a therapeutic success (when the treated individual's subjective condition was in fact an irreversible impairment of their already reduced capacity to understand and act).

Finally, it can be observed that modes of behaviour deemed disreputable by the context of reference have led psychiatry to introduce diagnostic categories of which there was probably no need, but which were considered legitimate by the scientific community. An emblematic case of mental illness registered by the DSM, but today highly debated as such, is that of the so-called ADHD (Attention Deficit Hyperactivity Disorder). As the label suggests, it is a condition characterised by the inability to concentrate and remain still and composed for a long time. It manifests itself mainly in school contexts, in which the child or young person who is unable to remain calmly receptive to lessons for long is (understandably) frowned upon by adults.

Many scholars have disputed that the diagnosis of ADHD is legitimate as such. However, of great concern to mental health scholars has been both the relative ease with which ADHD is diagnosed and the treatment with which it is treated (usually the administration of drugs such as Ritalin). Firstly, in fact, it is likely that even children who in the past would have been considered simply a bit agitated are diagnosed as suffering from ADHD; secondly, the taking of medical drugs by minors who do not in fact represent a danger to themselves or others should be considered an extreme case, given the inevitable side effects that such taking entails.

Notes

1 Hobsbawm, *The Age of Extremes*, 558.
2 Van Voren, *Soviet Psychiatric Abuse in the Gorbachev Era*, 187; see also Savelli and Marks, *Psychiatry in Communist Europe*.
3 American Psychiatric Association, *DSM-5_TR*, 101.
4 American Psychiatric Association, *DSM-5_TR*, 102.

5 Gabbard, *Psychodynamic Psychiatry*, 150.
6 Gabbard, *Psychodynamic Psychiatry*, 173.
7 Kraepelin, *Lehrbuch der Psychiatrie* 1896 and 1899 editions; see also Bleuler, *Dementia Praecox.*
8 Jung, *Psychology of Dementia Praecox.*
9 Bleuler, *Dementia Praecox*, 9.
10 Bleuler, *Dementia Praecox*, 463.
11 See this idea developed again in Smulevich, "Sluggish Schizophrenia", i.e. in a text written after the advent of Gorbachev; see also Smith and Oleszczuk, *No Asylum.*
12 Zajicek, "Soviet Madness"; Zajicek, "Soviet Psychiatry".
13 Koryagin, "Unwilling Patients".
14 Lavretsky, "The Russian Concept of Schizophrenia".
15 See, e.g., Van Voren, "Political Abuse of Psychiatry".
16 Savelli and Marks, *Psychiatry in Communist Europe.*
17 Zajicek, "Soviet Psychiatry".
18 See, e.g., Marx, *Economic and Philosophic Manuscripts of 1844.*
19 Zajicek, "Soviet Psychiatry".
20 Zajicek, "Soviet Madness".
21 Payne, *S. L. Rubinstein.*
22 Costa, *Psicologia sovietica.*
23 Gannushkin, *Clinical Aspects of Psychopathies.*
24 Kerbikov, *Selected Papers.*
25 Zajicek, "Soviet Psychiatry".
26 Suchareva, "The Soft Forms of Schizophrenia".
27 Melekhov, Shubina, and Kogan (eds.), *Schizophreniya.*
28 See Introduction.
29 Onians, *The Origins of European Thought.*

7 Shamanism and Arctic Hysteria

7.1 The Story of a Goldi Shaman

A 40-year-old Siberian shaman of the Nanai people told an ethnologist that his own vocation began with an illness. He had never, for the first 20 years of his life, thought about the possibility of becoming a shaman. None of his immediate family members were shamans, although elders had later told him that great shamans were among his ancestors. In his early 20s, he had begun to suffer terrible headaches and widespread pain throughout his body. Shamans had tried to heal him but in vain. Healing had only come as a result of his shamanic vocation and the possibility of performing *rituals* on himself. At first, he himself had been the only beneficiary of his own cures. Only later had he begun to cure others, also because "the profession of the shaman", he used to say, "is tiring, very tiring".[1]

The vocation had presented itself through the vision of a spirit guide:

> Once I was asleep on my sick-bed, when a spirit approached me. It was a very beautiful woman. Her figure was very slight, she was no more than half an arshin (71 cm) tall. Her face and attire were quite as those of one of our Gold women. Her hair fell down to her shoulders in short black tresses. Other shamans say they have had the vision of a woman with one half of her face black, and the other half red. She said: I am the 'ayami' of your ancestors, the Shamans. I taught them shamaning. Now I am going to teach you. The old shamans have died off, and there is no one to heal people. You are to become a shaman.[2]

The *àyami* went on to express her intention to become his wife (since she was now without a husband) and to help him by leading other spirits to him who would help him in the art of healing. If he obeyed her, much honour would be bestowed on him and people would bring him food without him having to procure it. If not, she would kill him – which definitely convinced the now candidate shaman, who, as far as he reported, was not initially inclined to follow the *àyami*.

DOI: 10.4324/9781003481249-8

From then on, the woman began to visit him frequently and to have sexual relations with him. The dwelling of the *àyami* was an isolated hut in which she lived all alone without any family. However, she changed her abode as often as her appearance, sometimes manifesting herself as an old woman and sometimes as a terrifying-looking wolf or even as a winged tiger. In the latter guise, she transported him to distant places inhabited by strange peoples, some consisting only of youngsters and others only of old inhabitants. On some occasions, both were transformed into tigers. Mircea Eliade comments:

> All these details of ecstatic journeys are most important. In North and Southeast Asia the Spirit-Instructor of young candidates for initiation appears in the form of a bear or a tiger. Sometimes the candidate is carried off into the jungle (symbol of the beyond) on the back of such an animal-spirit. People who turn themselves into tigers are initiates or "dead men" (which, in myths, is sometimes the same thing).[3]

The visits of the *àyami* had initially been very frequent and then had thinned out over time. In any case, he had left the now-initiated shaman three assistants: a panther, a bear, and a tiger, who visited him in his sleep and, above all, could be summoned whenever it was necessary to practise the shamanic art. If they were reluctant to manifest themselves, the *àyami* would compel them (she was powerful, but it seems that some spirits could sometimes resist even her).

During rituals, the shaman was penetrated by the *àyami* and other "auxiliary" spirits as would happen with steam or moisture. When she spoke, it was the *àyami* who spoke in her place. When she consumed offerings, it was she who ate. When she drank pig's blood (an act of exclusive shamanic pertinence), it was always she who drank it.

7.2 Shamanism and Psychopathology

If such a story were told by a modern-day Western European, no one would be willing to take the protagonist seriously. It is not entirely uncommon for someone to claim to have been chosen by a spirit guide and, penetrated by it, to be able to speak with its voice. Yet our culture regards him, at best, as a charlatan who pretends to possess such an ability in search of gullible people; at worst, a psychotic suffering from delusions, probably dangerous to himself and others. Delusions are technically defined today as "established false certainties, often concerning events experienced as if they had really happened".[4] Of course, however, the concept of "false certainty" cannot be understood in an absolute sense, but only with respect to the cultural and historical moment.

A little over a century ago, the possibility that mediums actually existed that could summon spirits and speak with their voices was accepted even by the most respected psychologists and scientists. William James, who in addition to being the father of pragmatism was one of the most respected empirical psychologists of his time, participated in séances and even joined the Theosophical Society, founded by the most famous medium of his time, Madame Blavatsky. James was just one of many intellectuals who "did not exclude" the idea that paranormal experiences could bring psychological and philosophical insights.[5] Jung, for example, dedicated his thesis to his cousin Hélène Preiswerk, a self-styled medium, with a fairly open attitude towards the latter's faculties.[6] Having then discovered that his cousin was faking everything, Jung did not lose heart and reversed the perspective he had begun to adopt, entitling his work *Psychology and Pathology of So-called Occult Phenomena*. It should not be forgotten that even today, in a non-minority part of Catholic circles, the belief persists that the possessed individual can speak with the voice of the possessing demon.

These circumstances alone should warn of the risk of "ethnocentrism" on the part of a culture that regards shamans as visionary madmen. Yet this has repeatedly occurred, as will be shown below. For the moment, it should be noted that there is a fundamental difference between a mentally ill person and a mystic such as a shaman:

> Regarded in the horizon of the *homo religiosus* [...] the mentally ill patient proves to be an unsuccessful mystic or, better, the caricature of a mystic. His experience is without religious content, even if it appears to resemble a religious experience, just as an act of autoeroticism arrives at the same physiological result as a sexual act properly speaking (seminal emission), yet at the same time is but a caricature of the latter because it is without the concrete presence of the partner.[7]

On the contrary, from the point of view of the Goldi culture and others like it, what we call mental illness must be considered a *necessary premise* and, in some ways, even an *occupational hazard* of the shaman. It can be considered a necessary premise because, in the initiation process of the shaman, the vocation coincides with a state of suffering. The Goldi shaman whose story was told went through a long period of physical suffering before seeing the spirit guide and being healed. This seems a wholly typical example. As one of the first scholars of shamanism wrote:

> Whether the vocation is hereditary or not, the shaman must be a capable, nay, inspired person. Of course, this is practically the same thing as saying that he is nervous and excitable, often to the verge of insanity. So long as he practises his vocation, however, the shaman never passes this verge. It often happens that before entering the calling, persons have had serious nervous affections. Thus a Chukchee female shaman, Telpina, according to her own statement, had been violently insane for

> three years, during which time her household had taken precautions that she should do no harm to the people or to herself.[8]

Moreover, full shamanic initiation did not represent a guarantee of achieved inner calm, if it is true that a Kelewgi shaman reacted by unsheathing his knife to a refusal to buy furs from a member of another tribe.[9] Initiation, in any case, necessarily involves steps that involve putting one's physical and mental health at risk, for instance through long periods of fasting and isolation.

The mythology of all times and all countries is filled with the recurrence in different forms of the theme of suffering connected to initiation or at any rate to the possibility of acquiring a higher state of consciousness: the various myths connected to the passage through the realm of the dead; those of magicians, often kings, thaumaturges but marked by an incurable wound; the blindness of Homer and of the soothsayers Nestor and Tiresias; the loss of an eye by Wotan; up to the legend imagined by Josef Knecht, protagonist of Hesse's *The Glass Bead Game*, about the impossibility of understanding the meaning of life if one has not been sufficiently ill.

Even the vocation of the Western psychoanalyst seems to arise from a condition of psychological suffering. Ellenberger argued that both Freud and Jung went through a "creative illness", i.e. a period of dangerous regression, which ended, however, with the conception of new and important theories.[10] The very idea of training analysis as a necessary requirement to become a therapist in turn is nothing but a *cure* for the future therapist. The Italian analyst Aldo Carotenuto, in several works, used the metaphor of a *ferita-feritoia* (wound-slit) to express the idea that only the first-person suffering of the analyst allows the understanding gaze on the suffering of the other. The association between psychoanalyst and shaman, based on the pathological condition, was object of interest also for the anthropologist Lévi-Strauss, who wrote: "a patient successfully treated by a shaman is in an especially good position to become a shaman in his own right, as we see today in the case of psychoanalysis".[11] Lévi-Strauss, moreover, believed that the shamanic therapeutic technique also had aspects in common with the psychoanalytic one:

> In psychoanalysis, abreaction refers to the decisive moment in the treatment when the patient intensively relives the initial situation from which his disturbance stems, before he ultimately overcomes it. In this sense, the shaman is a professional abreactor.[12]

A specific risk to mental health, however, is connected to the shamanic initiatory path. In order to become an Arctic shaman, one must have visions. However, if they are unable to conjure up visions of their own accord, but it is the visions that seize them without their will, they become a mere sufferer of *Arctic hysteria*.[13] According to this reading, Arctic hysteria would then be the pathological condition of the would-be shaman who becomes the victim of what would otherwise be a gift, if they were able to control it. It should be noted that, according to some of Mircea Eliade's sources, only the shamans of the far north, helped in this evidently by the extreme climate, would have been able to have visions spontaneously. The *sub-Arctic* shamans, on the other hand, would have needed to help themselves with drugs. Finally, the Arctic shaman would have been subject to another potential risk: that of falling ill if they did not practise their art frequently enough.[14] In summary, then: pathology would have constituted a condition prior to the moment of vocation; a risk during initiation; a further potential risk after initiation itself. It would not, however, have characterised the condition of the shaman as such.

Quite a few anthropologists who have described Arctic hysteria as a form of mental illness in the populations of the far north over the course of time have instead identified shamans as representatives of a generally male expression of this illness.[15] In women, rarely shamanic figures and instead more often subject to the same disease, the pathology has been connected with disorders of the female genital apparatus, or at least this was the interpretation of the anthropologist Jochelson.[16] The latter, applying categories from Western psychiatry and noting the analogy with the behaviour described as peculiar to the classical hysterics, chose for the first time to translate the terms used among the indigenous peoples of Siberia and Alaska (*pibloktoq*, *meryak*, and *menerik*), as "Arctic hysteria".

In fact, the link between shamanism and the pathological condition has been read in the most varied ways by Western interpreters, from the perspective that shamans are nothing more than "culturally accepted schizophrenics or neurotics" who exhibit dissociation and sexual and/or behavioural aberrations, as well as often paranoid thoughts of persecution; to the idea that shamans are some of the most intelligent, best adapted, creative and insightful members of their communities.[17]

It must be said that the more extreme views, which qualified shamans as merely psychotics[18] or epileptics subject to attacks of "high evil" ("*haut-mal*"), were presumably based on rough, unsystematic and impressionistic descriptions of their behaviour.[19] More recently it has been observed that there are differences between schizophrenic and epileptic attacks on the one hand and shamanic practices on the other, not only in terms of the "voluntary" nature of these states but also in terms of the "affective, perceptual and cognitive" correlates associated with them.[20]

7.3 Arctic Hysteria and Its Various Manifestations

There were no written descriptions of these diseases prior to the Arctic explorations at the end of the 19th century, although similar phenomena may have been encountered by Russian travellers a century earlier. There is therefore no evidence as to how far their first manifestations preceded the encounter with Westerners. However, one interpretation of the origin of Arctic hysteria links it to just such an encounter, outlining the view that many researchers believe that *pibloktoq* did not exist "until native peoples came into contact with European and American populations". Researchers who support this hypothesis believe that *pibloktoq* is a manifestation of "stress and despair" related to a cultural shock.[21]

In any case, the first mention of the term *pibloktoq* appeared in the West in 1892 by Josephine Diebitsch Peary, wife of the better-known explorer Robert Peary. She had noted in her diary the strange behaviour of a woman she had seen fidgeting in the open, before being led back to the igloo by her husband. Asked for an explanation from the natives, she was told that she was indeed *pibloktoq* – a term that on this first occasion she trivially translated as "crazy". Robert Peary, in turn, documented the observation of other cases in 1909.[22] The symptoms have since been described in a fairly similar, though not overlapping, manner for the different populations on either side of the Bering Strait. A person first becomes irritable and grumpy and tends to withdraw into themselves. When the attack starts, they begin to tear their clothes off, scream uncontrollably, hurl curses, break objects they find within reach, eat excrement, and engage in dangerous behaviour such as running naked in the polar frost or walking on thin icy surfaces.[23] In some cases, convulsions or comatose conditions may occur. In any case, they will tend to forget everything that happened during the attack.[24] While *pibloktoq* would be characterised by "an excessive paroxysmal state alternating with a condition of total exhaustion"; *meryak* by less intense "epileptic episodes or catalepsy"; *menerik*, on the other hand, "defined milder cases, characterised by easy excitability and susceptibility to the slightest noises, which triggered strong tremors".[25]

From the point of view of the natives, in its various manifestations Arctic hysteria would be considered a physical illness, which relatives and friends of the sick person regard quietly and without particular surprise, given the habit of the manifestation and since the prodromes of the attacks are characterised by the mood changes described above, which are rather easy to identify. Family members usually designate someone to take care of the sick person during the attack, so that he or she does not get hurt; in any case, they do not worry about it and simply wait for the sick person to return to normal.[26]

From the Western point of view, different causes have been hypothesised. Not even the label "Arctic hysteria" has been used univocally, replaced from time to time by "temporary insanity", "transient insanity", "frenzied dissociative neurosis", "shock and fear neurosis", "atypical culture-related psychogenic psychosis", "hysterical dissociation state".[27] According to Dick, the main interpretative approaches are (1) psychoanalytic, which focus on the influence of personality development on behaviour; (2) environmental, which emphasise the impact of climate, cold, light, and related factors; (3) nutritional, which emphasise the effects of minerals or vitamins, either in excess or deficiency of normal dosages; (4) interdisciplinary approaches, which attempt to synthesise possible psychological, environmental, biological and cultural factors. To these, we can add a fifth explanatory category, underrepresented in the literature, which emphasises cultural or social factors in the aetiology of *pibloktoq*.[28]

Historian Lyle Dick, however, has even gone so far as to propose the paradoxical conclusion that Arctic hysteria does not exist and has never existed but is the result of a purely cultural invention of the Western world. Even the term *pibloktoq* would not exist but would be the result of incorrect transcriptions by anthropologists.

In this light, the creation of Arctic hysteria would thus be seen as a Foucauldian phenomenon, the result of the Western characteristic tendency to classify reality into normal and pathological, which would end up comprehensively labelling Arctic populations within a "pathological cultural identity, of which the shaman would be representative and champion".[29]

7.4 The Story of Qaselid, the Sceptical Shaman

One should not think that the relationship with the shamanism of the Arctic peoples is linear and never marked by scepticism. Here is a singular case of conversion:

> Sandschejew had come to know a Buryat who, in his youth, had been an 'anti-shamanist'. But he fell ill and, after vainly seeking a cure (he even traveled to Irkutsk in search of a good doctor), he tried shamanizing. He was immediately cured, and became a shaman for the rest of his life.[30]

Above all, it should not be assumed that all shamans are unaware that their virtues as healers are due to suggestion. In this regard, the story of the shaman Qaselid, of Kwakiutl origin, narrated by Boas and later taken up and commented on for its significance by both Lévi-Strauss and Ellenberger, appears illuminating.[31]

Qaselid had always doubted the reality of shamans' powers, even more so after witnessing a solemn ceremony led by the shaman Making-Alive, at the end of which he healed a sick man by "extracting" a kind of bloody worm from his chest, which he claimed was "the disease". Unconvinced of the truth of Making-Alive's claims, Qaselid nevertheless immediately accepted the offer to become a shaman himself. He therefore began a course of instruction, in which his doubts were confirmed:

> His narrative recounts the details of his first lessons; a curious mixture of pantomime, prestidigitation, and empirical knowledge; including the art of simulating fainting and nervous fits, the learning of sacred songs, the technique of inducing vomiting, rather precise notions of auscultation and obstetrics; and the use of 'dreamers', that is, spies who listen to private conversations and secretly convey to the shaman bits of information

> concerning the origins and symptoms of the ills suffered by different people. Above all, he learned the *ars magna* of one of the shamanistic schools of the Northwest Coast: The shaman hides a little tuff down in a corner of his mouth, and throws it up, covered with blood, at the proper moment – after having bitten his tongue or having his gums bleed – and solemnly present it to his patient and the onlookers as the pathological foreign body extracted as a result of his sucking and manipulations.[32]

Qaselid's doubts had become certainties, but by this time his apprenticeship was known to all, and when the young Food-Owner had dreamed that he would be healed by him, Qaselid had decided to acquiesce, practising in turn the technique of the bloody wad. He achieved an initial great success, which earned him the sacred name of Qaselid and which he lucidly attributed to Food-Owner's firm belief in the dream about him. While visiting a Koskimo tribe, he had then witnessed a ceremony by local shamans to heal Woman-Made-to-Invite, the daughter of a chief. The local shamanic technique was much less refined than the Kwakiutl one: the Koskimo shamans only showed a bit of saliva as a "disease-object". In any case, Woman-Made-to-Invite had not been cured. Qaselid thought that, all things considered, his technique was a minor cheat. At least it showed something tangible. Offering to try it himself, Qaselid repeated the wad ceremony, and this time Woman-Made-to-Invite declared that she felt healed. In vain, the local shamans asked Qaselid to reveal his technique, and the aura of the great shaman grew stronger around him.

An elderly shaman, himself of considerable reputation, challenged him to a kind of competition to see who could heal the most patients. He too used an unrefined technique, simulating extracting an invisible object from the body of the sick. Qaselid triumphed in this case too, healing a woman who claimed to have been cured several times, but without success, by the elderly shaman. The latter, through the pain of defeat and the snub of not being able to have Qaselid's secret revealed to him, ended up going mad. Ellenberger writes:

> Qaselid continues to study the tricks of other shamans, while adding to his own therapeutic successes with the method of the bloody earthworm. At the end of the narrative, it is clear that he finds it more and more difficult to recognize the 'real' shamans from the quacks. He is sure only of one who is a 'real' shaman because he does not accept payment from his patients and because he has never been seen laughing; all others 'pretend to be shamans'. On the other hand, Oaselid reports his own successes without apparently remembering that he started his career with the intention to unmask the tricks that he now applies himself very successfully.[33]

Regardless of the possible exaggerations contained in Qaselid's tale, this curious character had started out with the idea of unmasking shamans and found himself in turn in the role of a valued shaman, in a spiral of suggestion and autosuggestion. Qaselid, in fact, "did not become a great shaman because he healed the sick: he healed the sick because he had become a great shaman".[34] Thus an individual dimension (the shaman's self-confidence), a relational dimension (the relationship established between healer and cured; in psychodynamic terms: the transference), and a collective dimension (the status recognised by the community) intersect in the shaman's abilities.

> The [shamanic] ceremony, in turn, can become efficient only within a psychological and sociological framework that includes: (1) The healer's faith in his own abilities, even if he knows that part of the technique depends on some kind of quackery. (2) The patient's faith in the healer's abilities, as shown in the case of Qaselid's first patient. (The success and reputation of a healer increase, of course, the public's faith in his abilities.) (3) The disease, the healing method, and the healer must all be acknowledged by the social group. The shaman is a member of an organization that has its training, its schools, its strict rules, its meeting places, its secret agents, as well as rivalries with other similar organizations.[35]

All this, however, would seem to describe the shamanic figures as performers or hypnotists who are substantially aware of being so, and who aim to keep their intentions and techniques all the more rigorously concealed, the more it is the mysterious and "supernatural" aspect of their activity that guarantees their effectiveness. This would tend to exclude any aspect of sincerity in their faith in spirit guides, in their vocation, and in initiatory procedures, which include, as mentioned above, experiences of visions and soul journeys outside the body. Here, too, there is a risk of a re-emergence of the Western ethnocentric attitude that, unwilling to believe in spirits, ends up completely doubting that one can believe in them in different cultural environments. Lévi-Strauss hypothesised that, in fact, one can postulate a possible *rational* belief on the part of the shaman in their own initiatory experiences. In certain primitive languages, according to the French anthropologist, specific terms refer to knowledge of the supernatural world through perception and others to that obtained through reasoning. The idea of having experienced initiation could therefore develop *ex post*:

> The native who becomes a shaman after a spiritual crisis conceives of his state grammatically, as a consequence to be inferred from the fact – formulated as real experience – that he has received divine guidance. From the latter he concludes deductively that he must have been on a journey to the beyond, at the end of which he found himself – again, an immediate experience – once more among his people.[36]

This formulation appears perhaps a little abstract and forced. However, it is not too far removed from the hypothesis that the shaman, having developed fantasies or experienced dreams of initiation, becomes convinced that such fantasies and dreams are real experiences because their culture conceives the possibility of them, and that belief is reinforced by the efficacy of their therapeutic efforts. The shaman, therefore, might as well simulate having visions as have the ability to use their fantasy and stop it, except to convince themselves that their fantasy can produce real supernatural events. They would then find themselves in a third condition between the person who fantasises and knows that they are only using imagination and the psychotic who is the victim of hallucinations (which are also the result of fantasising) because they have lost the sense of the boundary between the real and the unreal and they are unable either to initiate his visions or to stop them.

Notes

1 Eliade, *Shamanism*, 47.
2 Eliade, *Shamanism*, 72.
3 Eliade, *Shamanism*, 72.
4 Othmer and Othmer, *The Clinical Interview.*
5 Simon, *Genuine Reality*, 140.
6 Jung, *Psychology and Pathology of So-called Occult Phenomena.*
7 Eliade, *Shamanism*, 26.
8 Czaplinka, *Shamanism in Siberia*, 14.
9 Bogoras, "Chuckchee Mythology", 426.
10 Ellenberger, *The Discovery of the Unconscious.*
11 Lévi-Strauss, *Structural Anthropology*, 180.
12 Lévi-Strauss, *Structural Anthropology*, 181.
13 Eliade, *Shamanism.*
14 Sieroszewski, "Du chamanisme".
15 Beginning with Bogoras, "The Chuckchee Religion".
16 Jochelson, *Material Culture and Social Organisation of the Koryak.*
17 Throop and Dornan, "Psychopathology and Shamanism", 212.
18 Devereux, "Normal and Abnormal"
19 Fabrega and Silver, "Zinacanteco Shamans".
20 Throop and Dornan, "Psychopathology and Shamanism", 214.
21 Higgs, "Pibloktoq", 3.
22 Wallace and Ackerman, "An Interdisciplinary Approach to Mental Disorder among the Polar Eskimos".
23 Dick, "Pibloktoq".
24 Rhoades, "Cross-cultural Aspects of Trauma and Dissociation".
25 Montanari, "Il cibo dello sciamano", 268
26 Higgs, "Pibloktoq".
27 Dick, "Pibloktoq".
28 Dick, "Pibloktoq", 2.
29 Montanari, "Il cibo dello sciamano".
30 Eliade, *Shamanism*, 28.
31 Boas, "The Religion of the Kawkiutl"; Lévi-Strauss, *Structural Anthropology*; Ellenberger, *The Discovery of the Unconscious.*
32 Lévi-Strauss, *Structural Anthropology*, 175.
33 Ellenberger, *The Discovery of the Unconscious*, 12.
34 Lévi-Strauss, *Structural Anthropology*, 203.
35 Ellenberger, *The Discovery of the Unconscious*, 12.
36 Lévi-Strauss, *Structural Anthropology*, 179–180.

8 Amok

8.1 The (Literary) Story of Oceania's Mysterious Passenger

Stefan Zweig imagined, in a novella entitled *Amok*, the story that an anonymous European passenger tells on the ship Oceania to the narrator, describing a dramatic experience during his stay in Malaysia. The passenger describes his own behaviour as conditioned by the Malaysian environment, which leads many natives to fall into a pathology only known there, the amok:

> This is how it goes: a Malay, an ordinary, good-natured man, sits drinking his brew, impassive, indifferent, apathetic [...] just as I was sitting in my room [...] when suddenly he leaps to his feet, snatches his dagger and runs out into the street, going straight ahead of him, always straight ahead, with no idea of any destination. With his *kris* he strikes down anything that crosses his path, man or beast, and this murderous frenzy makes him even more deranged. He froths at the mouth as he runs, he howls like a lunatic [...] but he still runs and runs and runs, he doesn't look right, he doesn't look left, he just runs on screaming shrilly, brandishing his bloodstained *kris* as he forges straight ahead in that dreadful way. The people of the villages know that no power can halt a man running amok, so they shout warnings ahead when they see him coming – 'Amok! Amok!' – and everyone flees [...] but he runs on without hearing, without seeing, striking down anything he meets [...] until he is either shot dead like a mad dog or collapses of his own accord, still frothing at the mouth [...].[1]

The passenger from Oceania had not wielded a kris; he had not run into the street killing unfortunate "natives". However, he had been seized by an unbearable frenzy, which had led him down the road to ruin in a way he could never have foreseen. The protagonist of the story is a physician, forced by a scandal to leave his homeland, accepting an offer to become a colonial doctor in a remote place in Malaysia, where he had by then spent most of the time stipulated in the ten-year commitment he had signed up for. He had then become accustomed to limited contact with Westerners and the

DOI: 10.4324/9781003481249-9

possibility of satisfying his sexual appetites thanks to the humble complaisance of Malaysian girls, who seemed to feel honoured by the attentions of a white man.

One day, in his office, he had seen a strikingly beautiful English woman appear, who had asked him on the spur of the moment to procure an abortion for her, in exchange for exorbitant financial compensation. Three months pregnant, the woman had been waiting five months for her husband's return from the motherland. She was therefore looking for a professional who had no contact with her environment and had heard about the doctor because of an operation he had accidentally performed on a mutual acquaintance. The passenger from Oceania had refused the fee, hinting that only if she was physically available to him would he perform the illegal operation. He had been completely subjugated by her beauty and imperious manner, who despite her position of need looked down on him, strong in the knowledge of her social status and considerable financial means. The woman responded with a laugh of contempt and turned away, ordering him not to follow her.

At that point, the doctor's ordeal had begun. Initially paralysed by the contemptuous rejection of the counter-proposal, he had not managed to reach the woman before she left in her own car, but he had learned who she was and where she lived, thanks to the information that her driver had let slip with the locals in the meantime.

The doctor thus began a mad pursuit, willing by now to comply with the woman's dangerous demands without asking for anything in return. Thus, his account continues:

> Only an hour after that woman had entered my room, I had thrown my life away and was running amok, careering into empty space. I ran straight on, headlong [...] I arrived in the city at six in the evening, and at ten past six I was at her house asking to see her. It was [...] well, as you will understand, it was the most pointless, stupid thing I could have done, but a man runs amok with empty eyes, he doesn't see where he is going. The servant came back after a few minutes, cool and polite: his mistress was not well and couldn't see anyone.[2]

The eagerness to make himself available at all costs, which had prompted the doctor to look for the woman again in public situations, ended up getting him rejected again. A letter written to unconditionally offer his services had come back with an interlocutory reply, a request to wait. And the doctor waited: "I spent the day, just waiting, waiting, waiting [...] but waiting like a man running amok, senselessly, like an animal, with that headlong, direct persistence".[3] In the meantime, the woman had unluckily placed herself in the hands of a "mother", who had performed a clumsy abortion, putting her life at risk. Only too late had she called the doctor, who despite a night of effort could only surrender to the ineluctable: "I collapsed beside her bed [...] just as a man running amok falls senseless at the end of his frenzied career, his nerves broken".[4]

Zweig's literary imagination, therefore, juxtaposes the physical frenzy of the Malaysian with a bladed weapon with the mental frenzy of the Westerner, who virtually clutches a cutting tool in his hand, i.e. the surgeon's scalpel. Inducing the uncontrolled behaviour would always be the environment, the *genius loci*.

8.2 The Characteristics of Amok

The word *amok* or *amuk* originated in the context of the Bahasa Malaya language, spoken today by some 250 million people in Malaysia, Indonesia, Singapore, Brunei, southern Thailand, the Philippines – and also elsewhere, at least as a second language. Throughout this area, the term has been known for a long time and indicates the unique form of pathology vividly described in the first quotation from Zweig's novel. In one of the more succinct definitions, it is an "attack of savage rage" to which the Malay male is subject, the cause of which is "not known". In this state the amok runner "attacks blindly anyone he meets, often injuring and killing many people before being shot down".[5] Equally well known in the same linguistic milieu are the two derived words *mengamok/mengamuk* (indicating a violent angry attack that leads to indiscriminate killing, or fighting in battle with impetuosity, or even wreaking havoc) and *pengamok/pengamuk* (the person subject to amok).[6] The expression "to run amok" has steadily become a proverbial motto in Anglo-Saxon countries to express the frantic race for its own sake, without an apparently rational purpose; it is not at all unusual, for instance, for it to be written in a scientific article that cancer cells "run amok", to express their race towards replication.

Apparently, the first Westerner to offer a description of *amok* in a travel report was the Italian explorer Nicolò Conti in the 15th century, followed by the Portuguese Duarte Barbosa in 1516.[7] During Cook's stay in Malaya in the 1770s, one of his officers reported being made aware of at least one case of amok every week.[8] However, more in-depth observations of the phenomenon, which reported its widespread occurrence in Malaysia, date back to the 19th century, the time when the area was a British colony that was systematically exploited by the occupiers.

With an ethnocentric perspective, an English witness, Sir Thomas Stamford Raffles, expressed his amazement at the contrast between the instinctive aggressiveness of the Malaysians and their capacity for self-control and courtesy of manner, which led them to be "the most well-behaved savages of whom we have knowledge".[9] The Malays were portrayed as inclined to avenge any offence with the *kris* or the *parang* (both familiar, especially the first, to the reader of Joseph Conrad's Malaysian novels) and always went around armed, but rarely got physical. The *amok* would thus have been the expression of the unleashing of an aggressive drive latent in the social character of the people.

The clinical descriptions of the late 19th and early 20th century all seem rather homogeneous in describing the course of amok.[10] The first phase, the preamble of the outbreak, would be the condition of *sakit hati* ("heart full of pain" or "sick liver"), which can follow from several causes, such as an offence suffered, jealousy over a real or feared betrayal (which can give rise to paranoid ideation), sadness over a loss can trigger a phase of isolation, at first marked by feelings of shame and shyness (*maloe*), then by increasingly intense rumination, which is also characterised by aggressive responses to those who try to distract from it.

The second phase is characterised by a condition of progressive obnubilation, called in Malay *gelap mata* ("black eyes"), which leads to the phase of madness and violence: the *pengamok* grabs the first weapon in their hand (traditionally cold steel) and starts to run in a straight line and assault anyone who stands in their way. As in Zweig's account, word of the amok attack spreads to the surroundings through the screams of those who see it; the reaction can be one of flight as well as organisation, in order to block the attack. Apparently, the phenomenon was so common in the late 19th century that every Malaysian village was equipped with a specially designed contraption to block the *pengamok*: a long stick with a noose at the end. Killing the *pengamok* to prevent it from committing further murders was in any case common practice at the time. A Victorian traveller describes the general reaction of villagers to a *pengamok* by recounting that "men feel no more scruple about killing him in his frenzy than they would have in killing a man-eating tiger".[11]

The few survivors, at the time, ended up becoming slaves of the rajah.[12] The frequent death of the protagonists has led some interpreters to consider at least some cases of apparent amok as forms of suicide. Malay culture considered it unacceptable to take one's own life but did not hold the *pengamok* morally responsible for their acts.[13] However, this hypothesis seems to be disproved by statistics, which have recorded more cases of suicide than amok over time.[14] If the attack does not end with the death of the protagonist, there is a halt due to the loss of strength, which is followed by a kind of stupor that finally results in complete amnesia of the violent acts just committed (third phase).

Faced with the survivors, the attitude of the cultural context changed. Until the colonisation of Malaysia, the albeit vindictive local culture did not call for punishment of the *pengamok*, considering their behaviour completely independent of personal will. Under British jurisdiction, in the 19th century, the tendency was instead to impose the death penalty, reversing the view of the individual responsibility. In the course of the 20th century, however, amok began to be regarded as a form of psychopathology.

The phenomenon of amok, while becoming much rarer in Malaysia, eventually spread beyond the confines of the strictly Malay-speaking culture – as far as is known, only during the 20th century – involving other neighbouring nations such as Laos, Cambodia, the Philippines, and Vietnam. The spread of amok seemed to be epidemic in nature. In every nation where it first appeared, or where it reappeared after a period of dormancy, there was a rapid rise in the number of cases, generally concentrated in a specific province, and an equally rapid descent, to reach a low *plateau* or almost disappear. This is particularly evident in Laos and the Philippines. In Laos, the first case was recorded in 1959. There was a rapid increase in amok until 1966, with a clear epicentre in the Vientiane region, i.e. right where the first case occurred. Fewer and fewer cases were seen in the following years until the curve flattened out to a very low number. In the Philippines, amok appeared in 1947 and saw a rapid but rather modest increase in cases up to the number of five in 1953 and a rapid decline thereafter. Almost all cases involved members of the armed forces.[15]

The traditional form of attack has also varied. In addition to bladed weapons, there have been cases where the *pengamok* acted with a stick or even their bare hands, but also situations where guns, cars, or even grenades have been used.[16] The mode of weapon use also often seems to be characterised by an epidemic-imitative character. All Filipino soldiers used a gun in their crises, just as handy as a *kris* for the Malaysians. The first case of *pengamok* armed with a grenade occurred in Laos (at a time when it was certainly not difficult to procure weapons of war in that area) and all subsequent cases followed the same technique, such as the two cases recorded in Thailand in 1971, located in an area bordering Laos. This circumstance seems to confirm the observation that in every nation and in every ethnic group where the amok appeared, in the Far East, there seems to have been contact with a culture in which this phenomenon was present, following similar patterns. Apparently, those who used for the first time a means of offending other than the traditional cold steel offered grounds for a diagnosis of psychosis after the amok episode (if not before). Their emulators, on the other hand, do not seem to have shown signs of mental problems except during the attack.[17]

Forms of pathology have also been categorised that are akin to amok, although not entirely identifiable with it. Gimlette distinguished between "true" and "false" amok, describing the latter as a furious attack on a specific person, with conscious motives and without loss of memory.[18] It is not impossible that the distinction was a relative one and that in some cases it went from intentional murder to actual amok attack. One such case is recorded by an English colonial authority from the late 19th century, who recounts a certain Mamat, a 45-year-old imam, previously considered to be a calm and well-balanced person, who showed up one morning armed with a knife and spear at the home of his sister and brother-in-law. With the utmost apparent calm, Mamat apologised to both of them before inflicting mortal wounds on them. Having completed his armament with two more spears found in the same house, Mamat began to rampage in the vicinity, violently, uncontrollably, and randomly killing several other people, including small children, within a hundred metres.[19]

Manic behaviour similar to amok has also been attributed to physical causes, such as malaria and epilepsy. A form considered to be true amok seems to be linked to hallucinations, as a result of which one believes one is being attacked by ferocious beasts, so that the *pengamok* has the illusion of defending themselves rather than attacking. According to Van Loon, this would indeed be the typical form of amok manifestation.[20] One might observe that such an assertion is speculative in nature, since the *pengamok* hardly remembers what happened during the attack, provided they survive it. Van Loon, however, based his assertion on the following considerations: (a) some *pengamok* retained, as their last memory before the "black eyes" phase, the feeling of having been attacked; (b) many cases of "unconsciousness" were followed by the sheer act of fleeing or throwing themselves into the water; and (c) aggression did not seem to manifest itself until the person under attack encountered obstacles or attempts to stop it. Although this last assertion seems to be somewhat circular (how would aggression manifest itself with a weapon, if not against someone?), it cannot be ruled out that Van Loon's assertion was at least valid for the manifestations of amok in the period and environment he observed (Batavia, then capital of the Dutch Indies). Just as it cannot be excluded that different forms of dissociation developed alongside amok. Van Loon records cases of mental confusion without hallucination and rage, resulting in the most diverse forms of behaviour: denuding, dancing, setting fire to one's house, or procuring various forms of self-mutilation.

As the definition above specifies, amok has been unanimously considered a syndrome that affects, in its original setting, only men (generally between the ages of 25 and 50). Almost exclusively women are instead affected by *lattah* or *latah*, which is therefore generally considered the female counterpart of amok, with which it has in common the sudden onset, the transient loss of consciousness, and the amnesia that generally follows the attack. Its expression, however, is very different: it starts as an exaggerated reaction to a stimulus that produces "fright" and manifests itself as a sudden impulse to burst into vulgar and obscene speech, a compulsive tendency to imitate someone else's movements, and an equally intense compulsion to obey orders that are given.[21] It was Gilles de la Tourette himself who observed that *lattah* had similarities with the syndrome that was later named after him.[22] However, the conclusion of the attack seems much easier. According to Van Loon, it was even sufficient to speak in a quiet voice without an imperative tone to bring a person out of the condition of *lattah*.[23] No wonder, then, that in the course of time there has been much discussion about the possibility of this being a simulated behaviour rather than a genuine pathology.[24]

8.3 Amok and the West

Between the end of the 19th and the beginning of the 20th century, the main diagnostic categories of Western psychiatry traced mental disorders to one of the following categories: (1) hysteria, epilepsy, hystero-epilepsy;

(2) *dementia praecox*, schizophrenia or psychosis in general; (3) physical illnesses of various kinds, specifically (4) lesion or alteration of the brain area; (5) melancholia/depression; and (6) mental automatism/dissociation. As evidence of how amok resists a traditional classification, one can see how attempts have been made over time to bring it into each of these categories.

Kraepelin, who was for a long time the only one to frame amok in a psychiatry diagnostic manual, considered it to be an epileptoid form,[25] but we have already seen how the connection with epilepsy seems implausible. Hysteria, which is more rarely associated with amok,[26] has instead been proposed as an explanation for lattah.[27] Swettenham suggested that all *pengamok* were psychotic[28] and more recent authors also seem to lean towards this explanation,[29] which Kraepelin did not exclude a priori. However, if the diagnosis of "traditional" psychosis appears legitimate in some cases, it seems to contrast with the descriptions of the psychological condition of many *pengamok* after the end of the attack, and apparently before it. Moreover, Van Loon, who had observed several cases of amok, qualified the moment of the attack as psychotic delirium but considered its nature to be completely different from that known in the Western European world.[30]

Ellis, based on the *sakit hati* condition preceding the attack, leaned towards a depressive tendency,[31] as did ethnologist James Logan.[32] But the very idea of *sakit hati*, which refers to a condition of physical malaise that the Malays themselves believed to be the cause of amok, was considered a clue to a possible organic cause, as hypothesised by Van Loon;[33] and some autopsies reported slightly altered brain conditions.[34] Another widespread belief among the Malays, that of a possible transient demonic possession, was also considered plausible, at least by the English judge who imposed a death sentence on a particularly heinous *pengamok*. The hypothesis of the heredity of amok was taken into consideration[35] especially at the time when the concept of the progressive degeneration of psychopathology between one generation and the next was achieving great cultural success.[36]

The link with dissociation is even sanctioned by the DSM-IV-TR, which frames amok, in the context of "culture-bound syndromes", as a "dissociative episode characterized by a period of brooding followed by an outburst of violent, aggressive, or homicidal behaviour directed at people and objects".[37] This definition, which is in fact rather vague, allows it to be likened to other syndromes characterised by agitation and extemporaneous aggression, such as *mal de pelea* in Puerto Rico or *iich'aa* of the Navajo, which have been in turn likened to Arctic hysteria,[38] with which amok certainly has little in common. It should be noted, incidentally, that amok was removed from the list of "culture-bound syndromes" in the DSM-5, without the circumstance being reported in any way.[39] One can only assume that the task force of the new DSM considered the phenomenon to have disappeared or become irrelevant.

Teoh and Schmidt, Hill, and Guthrie have argued that, like its phenomenology, the psychological causes of amok have also changed over time.[40] This conclusion, which Imai and collaborators also arrive at in a very recent review,[41] however attractive it may be to the author of this book, is nevertheless risky. It could in fact merely reflect a change in observer bias over time.[42] There is no doubt, for instance, that the word amok has taken on different meanings, being applied more and more broadly. Hatta, for example, has observed that today in Malaysia and among the different Malay-speaking populations of Southeast Asia, the word amok does not necessarily involve the meaning of "mental insanity"; rather, it has acquired a myriad of meanings, from the child throwing a tantrum to the violent attack of a soldier, and also to animals, such as the elephants who are taken by the amok destroying plantations or the amok of the swarm of bees whose hive has been damaged with a stick by children.[43]

The broadening of meaning is also expressed through the metaphorical use of the term outside the original cultural context: if someone (as mentioned above) writes that tumour cells *run amok* (proliferate in the grip of amok), one cannot obviously conclude either that amok is expressed today as tumour, or that amok can be subject to some cells and no longer just the human being with their mind. Thus, while it is possible that amok has changed over time, it is equally possible that it identifies a different pathology today than it did a hundred and fifty years ago; or that the same term encompasses different pathologies today.

Some authors questioned the idea that the person subjected to amok had never shown signs of imbalance before the withdrawal phase, just before the murderous attack, stating that in a Western context families would certainly have entrusted the potential *pengamok* to psychiatric services. This belief, however, seems to have been disproved over time by the phenomena of *serial killers* and *rampage killers*, recorded in the West especially since the last decades of the 20th century. The former expression indicates persons who kill numerous victims, one at a time and often over a rather long time span, choosing them for certain common characteristics (e.g. blonde girls and sex workers), usually following a precise ritualisation.[44] Expression and definition, which only originated in the 1970s, have now been introduced even into pop culture by an endless number of novels, films, and television series, which have described such figures by depicting them as generally inscrutable to families and acquaintances.[45] The apparent unsuspiciousness a priori seems to be a common element of the serial killer and the rampage killer, who instead kills several victims in one event but one at a time, usually with firearms. He differs in this respect both from the classical mass murderer (who has no direct contact with the victims and generally uses an explosive) and from the homicidal-suicide, who is primarily driven by religious motivations.[46]

The rampage killer is of particular interest here because it has not only been approached but also identified with amok in recent times. Schmidtke

Schaller and Miller collected dozens of newspaper articles published in Germany and the United States in the 1990s in which the word amok was used to describe cases of multiple murders with firearms, in which the victims seemed to be chosen at random, and in any case had no personal relationship with the killer.[47] In the same contribution, it was pointed out that the distribution of the events from the space-time point of view showed irregularities. Some rampage killers seemed to initiate a sort of trend, generating followers who would imitate the killings and the killing technique, localised mainly in a neighbouring geographical area. It is therefore appropriate to distinguish between the characteristics of the leaders and those of the followers.

Collins conducted a micro-sociological analysis of the best-known rampage killer figures who have come onto the scene over the last three decades.[48] This analysis seems to reveal how the Western rampage killer's affinity with the classical Malay *pengamok* is very limited. In fact, the latter does not at all seem to be prey to a sudden impulse, but calmly plans the place of the killings, gathering the weapons he will use. He plans a specific and paradoxical ritualisation (think of the title of Michael Moore's documentary *Bowling for Columbine*). He often utilises a particular dress code for the performance of his action, intended to mark his distance and difference from the predestined victims (e.g. black clothes, a camouflage suit, or even a police uniform in the infamous case of Anders Breivik).

The theatre of action and the victims have a symbolic value. For instance, it can be political in the narrow sense (in Breivik's case), or broader (schools, repeatedly hit by American students). Finally, the rampage killer tends to surrender without putting up any particular resistance to the forces of law and order. He does not lose control of his actions and prefers to allow himself to be stopped than to lose his life in an attempt to perpetrate new murders. In the case of the followers, which Collins does not seem to have considered very much, the symbolic element of the killings may in some cases be missing, replaced by purely formal imitation – even if the Internet has long been familiar with the figure of the "lone wolf", who becomes part of a vast network of people who share extremist ideas and plan politically motivated multiple murders.[49] However, the followers still retain the elements of "cold" preparation, starting with the precise choice of clothes in which to carry out their deed.[50]

Notes

1 Zweig, *Amok*, 21.
2 Zweig, *Amok*, 21.
3 Zweig, *Amok*, 27.
4 Zweig, *Amok*, 33.
5 Van Loon, "Amok and Lattah".
6 Hatta, "A Malay Crosscultural Worldview".
7 Spores, *Running Amok*.
8 Teoh, "The Changing Psychopathology of Amok".

9 Raffles, *The History of Java*, 532.
10 See, e.g. Ellis, "The Amok of the Malays"; Gimlette, "Notes on a Case of Amok".
11 Bird, *The Golden Chersonese*, 357.
12 Ellis, "The Amok of the Malays".
13 Kua, "Amok in Nineteenth-Century British Malaya History".
14 Westermeyer, "On the Epidemicity of Amok Violence".
15 Westermeyer, "On the Epidemicity of Amok Violence".
16 Schmidt, Hill, and Guthrie, "Running Amok".
17 Hatta, "A Malay Crosscultural Worldview".
18 Gimlette, "Notes on a Case of Amok".
19 Swettenham, *Malay Sketches*.
20 Van Loon, "Amok and Lattah".
21 Kenny, "Paradox Revisited".
22 Goetz and Klawans, "Gilles de la Tourette on Tourette Syndrome".
23 Van Loon, "Amok and Lattah".
24 Winzeler, *Latah in Southeast Asia*.
25 Kraepelin, "Psychiatry in Java".
26 Westermeyer, "On the Epidemicity of Amok Violence".
27 Van Loon, "Amok and Lattah".
28 Swettenham, *Malay Sketches*; Swettenham, *The Real Malay*.
29 See, e.g., Kua, "Amok in Nineteenth-Century British Malaya History".
30 Van Loon, "Amok and Lattah".
31 Ellis, "The Amok of the Malays".
32 Logan, "Malay Amoks and Piracies".
33 Van Loon, "Amok and Lattah".
34 See, e.g., Swettenham, *Malay Sketches*.
35 See, e.g., Ballard, "Letters, Notes, and Answers".
36 Pick, *Faces of Degeneration*.
37 APA, *DSM-IV-TR*, p. 899
38 Boindala et al., "Culture and Psychiatry".
39 APA, *DSM-5*.
40 Teoh, "The Changing Psychopathology of Amok"; Schmidt, Hill, and Guthrie, "Running Amok".
41 Imai, Ogawa, Okumiya, and Matsubayashi, "Amok: a Mirror of Time and People".
42 A phenomenon, moreover, already explicitly noted by Winzeler, *Latah in Southeast Asia*.
43 Hatta, "A Malay Crosscultural Worldview", 508.
44 Schmid, *Natural Born Celebrities*.
45 Hodgkinson, Prins, and Stuart Bennett, "Monsters, Madmen… and Myths".
46 Collins, "Micro-sociology of Mass Rampage Killings".
47 Schmidtke, Schaller, and Miller, "Imitation of Amok and Amok-suicide".
48 Collins, "Micro-sociology of Mass Rampage Killings".
49 Innamorati and Rossi, *La rete dell'odio*.
50 Schmidtke, Schaller, and Miller, "Imitation of Amok and Amok-suicide".

9 Hikikomori

9.1 The Story of Masuko-san

At the age of 16, Masuko-san begins to have difficulties at school and misses days. The parents soon realise that their son needs professional help and contact a specialised therapist, Takeshi Watanabe. Masuko-san, however, does not seem willing to talk about his problems and gradually locks himself in his room, only to come out to eat and go to the toilet. His life takes place at night behind the door of his room, in silence. He does not use telephone, television, or computer. The parents are bewildered. They end up leaving a tray with something to eat in front of the closed door so that Masuko-san can take it out to eat when he wants to and put it back when he is finished.

Takeshi Watanabe has already seen other Japanese youths practicing *hikikomori* and explains to the astonished parents that they must wait for Masuko-san to open the door, metaphorically and physically. Watanabe begins to wait, at regular times, in front of Masuko-san's door. For a long time, the door remains closed.

Finally, Watanabe is let in, but this does not yet mean the beginning of a verbal dialogue. Watanabe feels that he has to go along with Masuko-san's timing. He finds, in this, the support of Masuko-san's mother, who leaves Watanabe free to follow his strategy. Watanabe knows that in such cases a direct approach rather than helping the young hikikomori can push him into a definitive and irreversible closure. He enters the room and waits in silence. His presence must first be tolerated and then accepted. Sometimes the two simply sleep next to each other on the tatami mat in Masuko-san's room.

After a year of almost complete silence, Watanabe manages to introduce music into the relationship. It is part of his standard technique in treating young hikikomori. Masuko-san loves music. Together Watanabe and Masuko-san listen to medieval music, jazz, and finally also Western classical music. From the complete void, emotions gradually emerge. Some sporadic dialogue also begins, but Watanabe feels he reaches Masuko-san, behind his silence, mainly by listening to new music. It is classical music that seems to be the harbinger of a sort of slow path out of the young hikikomori's inner silence. Orff's *Carmina Burana* and Beethoven's *Fifth Symphony* (especially

DOI: 10.4324/9781003481249-10

the second and third movements) mark moments of particular intensity. But the piece that seems to captivate the young man completely is a track from Puccini's *Turandot*, the famous "Nessun dorma" sung by Luciano Pavarotti, made famous all over the world by the "Three tenors" concert in 1990. Paradoxically, neither Watanabe nor his patient knows the meaning of the words of "Nessun dorma", which nonetheless capture Masuko-san's inner state: "Even you, oh Princess/In your cold room/Watch at the stars/That tremble with love/And with hope…".

Twenty-four months of silence and music passed, with rare moments of verbal exchanges, until Masuko-san recalls an episode that happened to him when he was ten years old and tells it to his therapist. He was riding his bicycle to his school, when he was seized by a panic attack, fell to the ground, and lived for a while with the conviction that he would never get up again, that he would die there. The panic attack, however, had passed just as suddenly as it had come and had been repressed from his mind for eight whole years. He had not even told his parents about it.

Is that the distant origin of his withdrawal? He does not know (although anyone who reads his story inevitably thinks it more than likely). Is there another reason he can identify as the trigger for the withdrawal? He does not know. How did he feel when he started locking himself in his room? Not even that Masuko-san could say. Nor would he be able to say it at the end of his therapy. The most precise thing he can remember is that he had felt the need to *rest*, but precisely why, he cannot make that clear to himself or others.

Masuko-san and Watanabe continue to see each other, week after week. Month after month. Year after year. At the age of twenty-three, Masuko-san's mother decides to give him a puppy dog, which in its own way helps to bring the young man out of isolation. The puppy not only breaks the silence of the closed room but also needs to go outside, providing an opportunity for contact, however sporadic, with the world around him. After another five years of steady yet incredibly slow progress, Masuko-san is finally ready to return to society. Watanabe gives him one last appointment at a coffee shop. Reaching there, Watanabe finally proves to Masuko-san something that had seemed absolutely impossible to him for years: he can leave home alone and join someone else in a crowded place during the day. Watanabe parts ways from him.

He does not see him again until seven years later, when Carla Ricci, an Italian anthropologist, asks Watanabe to meet a hikikomori patient he treated. She will be the one to translate the lyrics of "Nessun dorma" into Japanese for the young man, revealing to an astonished Masuko-san how the words refer to the loneliness of two people, a loneliness that is precious to both of them but a prelude to a contact with the other, to a union, which represents the decisive step in their lives. Masuko-san, meanwhile, completed his studies, graduating in philosophy. He then found a job as an estate agent. He works even seven days a week away from home meeting clients, to whom he shows deep empathy. The agency is very satisfied with his work. Masuko-san eventually moved hundreds, even thousands of kilometres away from his home: he travelled in distant countries without speaking any language other than Japanese. Masuko-san expresses himself in gestures and always manages to make himself understood.

This is how Masuko-san describes his and others' teenage experience:

> During their teenage years, young people find themselves crossing a deep valley on a rope, like tightrope walkers. Most of them are good tightrope walkers and walk over it without thinking about it and arrive on the other side in a normal time; but some of them think about being on the rope all the time and are overcome with panic, can no longer move and refuse to continue to reach the other side. This is what young hikikomori feel.[1]

Masuko-san does not regret the period of complete isolation and, on the contrary, says he is convinced that it was a necessary moment in his life, a formative transition phase in his existential journey. In any case, Masuko-san is one of the rare examples of hikikomori where a complete remission of symptoms can be observed even after a rather long follow-up.

9.2 Hikikomori and Japan

The birth and spread of hikikomori might initially have appeared to be a typical example of a "transient mental illness" in the sense described by Hacking. Hikikomori was born at a fairly precise moment in history (the 1980s) and in an equally precise geographical area (Japan). It is described and explained by researchers as a phenomenon linked to a particular culture. It is also treated on site (*when* it is treated) in ways that appear unique to the eyes of the *gaijin*, the strange white-skinned human beings that we are to the Japanese. Masuko-san's experience, which began with years of silence, may be more of a rule than an exception. Hikikomori is often not even treated, for the simple reason that there seems to be no way to open a dialogue of any kind, not only with a therapist but also with the parents. There are no elements, however, to establish the *transience* of the hikikomori epidemic, because it is still widespread and our historical perspective is too close to assess the issue. Furthermore, for some years now, cases of hikikomori have also been reported in several other countries around the world.

The condition of hikikomori describes people who decide to voluntarily confine themselves in their rooms, refusing any form of physical contact with the outside world. The original definition proposed by psychiatrist Tamaki Saito, who first described the phenomenon and coined the term *hikikomori*, was the following:

> A state that has become a problem by the late twenties, that involves cooping oneself up in one's own home and not participating in society

> for six months or longer, but that does not seem to have another psychological problem as its principal source.[2]

Saito explained that the choice of identifying the upper age limit rather high was linked to the prolongation of adolescence in today's affluent society, when one can still feel like a "kid" even towards the end of the third decade of life. The expression "at least six months", on the other hand, met criteria of uniformity with respect to the DSM, where it often represents the minimum time of duration of symptoms to allow for a specific diagnosis. When, for example, a patient is considered to be diagnosed with schizophrenia, a personality disorder, or a phobia, the practitioner must check whether the specific symptoms correspond to the DSM description, but also bear in mind that these symptoms must have manifested themselves "over a period of at least six months".

The six-month condition, however, also reflected a functional criterion for Saito. A lower threshold (e.g. three months) could risk being over-inclusive, unnecessarily worrying families of young people who needed, perhaps, only a brief period of introspection; a higher threshold (e.g. one year) would allow greater diagnostic certainty but instead presented the risk of too late a demand for therapy (and much greater difficulties in treatment) on the part of the relatives. Subsequent studies tend instead to consider a period of three months sufficient for diagnosis, precisely with a view to early therapeutic intervention.[3]

Other symptoms were, however, considered by Saito to be typical of hikikomori: inversion of the day-night rhythm (night-time activity and daytime rest), excessive shyness, possible episodes of violence towards the parents (almost one in five cases, according to later reports), later possible addiction to the Internet. Suicide fantasy is another symptom often present in cases of hikikomori. Young people often go so far as to imagine how they will take their own life, down to the smallest details of the ritual that is to be performed. That suicide is carried out, however, is possible but rather rare. As if the hikikomori lacked the willpower for any decisive change in their existence.[4]

Saito notes that when social withdrawal persists, the young hikikomori also manifests an increasing exaltation of typically adolescent aspects of the personality, such as a tendency towards narrow-mindedness and inflexibility in pursuing one's own ideas. This is also reflected in the difficulty of admitting to having to ask for help. At this point, however, Saito seems to contradict himself: "The majority of hikikomori cases do not choose on their own to keep living that way just because they want to. They want more than anyone else to escape from their withdrawn situation, but they simply are not able to do so".[5] It is not entirely clear, therefore, whether Saito considers the symptoms *ego-syntonic* or *ego-dystonic*; that is, whether the hikikomori views them positively (as a suitable existential solution for him) or rather suffers from them and would like to get rid of them. Subsequent epidemiological studies have shown that 78% of Japanese hikikomori consider their condition problematic and would like to overcome it.[6] In any case, Masuko-san's attitude is the one that prevails. Establishing a therapeutic alliance, i.e. a mutual cooperation between patient and therapist, in cases of hikikomori is a long and problematic process.

The hikikomori's communication with family members may be so limited that it sometimes consists, as in Masuko-san's case, in simple pick-up and return of a tray with food necessary for survival, placed by the parents in front of the closed door. Occasionally, specific requests may be made to family members, which the hikikomori expect to be perfectly met. For instance, if they want a new hi-fi system, they may demand that it has carefully listed technical features. It would not be strange for failure to comply with these requests to trigger thoughtless reactions on the part of the hikikomori.

With people outside the family circle, the standard communication of the hikikomori may be entirely absent or limited to the virtual world. However, in recent times, it has been proposed to distinguish between *hard-core* and *soft-core* hikikomori. The latter might occasionally leave the house and exchange a few words with others;[7] the chosen place to spend one's daily life might then be, for instance, an internet café location rather than one's own room.

There are no signs, on the part of the young hikikomori, of a sense of responsibility for their actions. Sometimes some of them may manifest creativity. Sometimes they come out of their condition and find, like Masuko-san, a suitable place in the real world. In some cases, an underlying family conflict is present, but it is not a necessary condition for hikikomori.[8]

The term hikikomori comes from the Japanese verbs *hiku* and *komoru*. *Hiku* means to retreat, to pull back, to secure a safe place. *Komoru* means to hide, to shut oneself in, and refers to something difficult to see. According to Takeshi Watanabe, to translate the word would be to refer to three different English words implying the concept of "withdrawal": *to withdraw*, which indicates a defensive retreat, *to shut in*, which characterises a complete closure, and *to retreat*, which suggests reflection ("retreat" is also the word used to identify spiritual withdrawal).[9] In fact, many young people may begin self-isolating as a kind of temporary meditative retreat and perhaps would not even begin their retreat if they imagined the risk of excluding themselves from human contact for years.[10] Many others become hikikomori as a reaction to a particular experience. Others finally suffer from other mental illnesses. Some scholars have distinguished in this regard between *primary* and *secondary* hikikomori. The primary one would not involve the possible diagnosis of other psychiatric disorders. The secondary one would be the epiphenomenon of depression, schizophrenia or other psychopathologies usually classified in the DSM.[11] It has also been suggested that it is possible to distinguish four types of hikikomori: *alternative*, based above all on the non-acceptance of social norms; *reactionary*, characterised by unfavourable contexts in the school and family environment and often linked to a specific, traumatic, triggering event; *resignation*, consisting of the abandonment of competition in society; and *chrysalis-like*, in which anxiety about approaching adulthood prevails and a closure aimed at suspending awareness of the passage of time.[12]

According to an official survey carried out in Japan in 2016, 541,000 Japanese between the ages of 17 and 39 were diagnosed as hikikomori, of whom more than a third had been in this condition for at least seven years. Given that the previous government survey, dating back to 2010, recorded 696,000 cases, the phenomenon, although impressive, seems to be on the way down. However, it must be kept in mind that the figure excludes those in their 40s (among whom the phenomenon seems to be increasingly widespread today) and those who are in a hybrid condition, characterised for example by occasional trips out of the house with the family, so that the criterion of complete six-month isolation that the Japanese Ministry of Health, Labour and Welfare tends to apply, in order to contain the seriousness of the phenomenon, is not strictly verified.[13] Again, ministerial data dating back to 2009 revealed that the average age of hikikomori was around 32 and a half years. A more flexible estimate raises the number of hikikomori in Japan to the impressive figure of one million.[14]

In 90% of the cases treated by Saito, before turning into hikikomori, young people had progressively stopped going to school.[15] His conclusion was that non-attendance at school was an almost necessary, but fortunately not sufficient, preamble of hikikomori. It seems peculiar that, according to recent data from the OECD, Japanese 15-year-olds are the ones who miss the fewest days of school without justification among all the countries for which data exist: only 2% of them would have missed at least one school day. Paradoxically, however, almost 2% of upper secondary students end up skipping school regularly and more than 5% drop out before finishing.[16]

The causes of the emergence of this phenomenon have been attributed to a number of typical characteristics of Japanese society, to the dismay of local psychiatrists.[17] In Japan, the pressure to succeed in school and work, which is sensitive throughout the capitalist world, is particularly strong. Everyone is expected to go above and beyond their formal duties. Kenji Kawamoto's images of young Japanese men collapsing, exhausted by work fatigue, and even falling asleep in the street at the end of the working day are now legendary. Some companies require a total commitment on special occasions, which ends up recruiting the employee to the workplace. The case of specialists in video game software subject to continuous updating has turned this tendency into the work standard. Japan has experienced, especially at the height of its economic expansion in the 1980s, a phenomenon that constitutes the mirror opposite of hikikomori, that of death related to the excessive amount of work effort. The technical vocabulary introduced the words *karoshi*, death from the physical consequences of overwork, and *karojisatsu*, suicide from overwork.[18]

If the typical hikikomori candidate is the eldest male or only son of well-off families and high culture, this is presumably because it is on him that the highest expectations are generally focused. He is often the one for whom the family has already set a career, which is very likely to consist in replacing the father, especially if he is the head of a small or large company.[19] In general, the ratio of hikikomori men to hikikomori women is 9:1, and the latter tend to re-enter society more quickly.[20] To social pressures, the future hikikomori succumbs but is afraid of family and social judgement. Shame drives him to close the door of his room. The gesture, in Japanese culture, represents something absolutely paradoxical and inconceivable, for a number of reasons. The traditional Japanese home has no closed doors. Until relatively recently, the rooms of all houses were opened and closed by moving panels. "A house like a bellows!", Pinkerton exclaimed when visiting his future home in Puccini's *Madama Butterfly*. Instead, it happened that the only closed room in the house was the one where, in a culturally shared custom, the family member who showed signs of madness was confined for the rest of his or her life.[21]

If it is family pressures that drive withdrawal, it is family characteristics that enable it. The maternal role seems to be very significant in this respect:

> In Japan, the mother-child relationship is born and consolidated through what is called *amae*: a form of sweetness that belies a sweet dependence [...] The mother's behaviour is one of complete indulgence towards her son, overprotective and particularly indulgent [...] However, these are peculiarities that weaken the son since, as he grows up, he will absorb the awareness of his mother's goodness, of her sacrifice, and will develop a feeling of obligation towards her [...] and a dysfunctional bond is created.[22]

The hyper-protective mother figure is matched by an often absent father, absorbed as he is by work commitments.[23] Faced with the choice of social withdrawal, the family is, on the one hand, unsettled by the failure to respect an implicit code, on the other hand, incapable of intervening, whilst paradoxically going along with the situation, especially through the function of the mother.[24] In fact, one of the forms of intervention considered most important and effective in Japan consists in informing families, in order to enable them to deal with the problem rather than endure it, astonished as they are in almost all cases by behaviour contrary to any traditional code.[25]

9.3 Hikikomori Outside Japan

If the hikikomori phenomenon has gradually started to spread outside Japan, this is presumably because at least some of the characteristics of Japanese society are also (partly) present in different socio-cultural contexts. Among such characteristics, Li and Wong identify in particular a rigid education system, irregular employment opportunities, limited or rather downward tending social mobility, and the spread of social networks and online games.[26]

A life devoid of physical contact with the outside world has been made more attractive by the possibility of virtual contacts and the increasing variety of time use through technology. Indeed, in Japan, the emergence of hikikomori precedes the Internet boom while in the West it follows it. Kato and co-workers define hikikomori as an indicator of the emergence of a possible pandemic of psychological problems linked to the expansion of the global phenomenon of hyper-connectedness.[27]

In South Korea, where, out of a population of 50,000,000, there are an estimated 300,000 hikikomori (0.6% of the total), it seems that the strongest impetus for the increase in their numbers is due to online gambling addiction.[28] The example of South Korea may question the idea that simply removing the young person from their room would be the correct therapeutic move. South Koreans, in fact, are subject to compulsory conscription, but this does not seem to affect their tendency towards self-enclosure.

Some scholars tend to differentiate not only the causes but also the phenomenology of Japanese hikikomori from the rest of the world:

> The most important thing [...] is to identify it not as a rigid status of the person, as is currently the case in Japan, but rather as a dynamic and gradual condition. Hikikomori can then be interpreted as a drive for physical isolation, continuous over time, triggered as a reaction to the excessive pressures of realisation, typical of economically advanced capitalist societies.[29]

However, cross-national research conducted in Japan, India, Korea, and the United States seems to indicate similar psychological and social characteristics among hikikomori and equally similar preferences with respect to possible psychotherapeutic treatment.[30] On the other hand, a Spanish study argues for the general comorbidity of Iberian hikikomori with other forms of psychopathology.[31] In other words, it would be other mental illnesses that trigger symptoms that are a posteriori defined as hikikomori. The explicit conclusion is that this would be a new label to define pre-existing pathologies. If people suffering from depression lock themselves in their room, they are people suffering from depression and not something else.

Conversely, there are those who try to prove that hikikomori had existed outside Japan for some time, but had not yet been recognised as a specific syndrome. When the term had recently entered the international vocabulary, the Japanese psychiatrist Kato sent descriptions of two clinical vignettes of hikikomori to colleagues in various countries, asking them if they knew of any similar cases in their homeland. Positive responses came from all the other countries involved in the study, including (besides Japan and Korea) India, Bangladesh, Iran, Taiwan, Thailand, Australia and the United States.[32]

A common characteristic that is evident among the nations in which hikikomori is more widespread or seems to be at greater risk of spreading, consists in the coexistence of a fair degree of affluence and the prolonged cohabitation of young adults with their parents. Saito argues that this is precisely why in Spain and Italy, where such cohabitation affects 70% of adolescents and post-adolescents, the presence of hikikomori is particularly felt.[33] In the UK there are practically none, but there are at least 250,000 homeless young people. Youth distress is still present, but its results would have to be sought on the streets, rather than in heated and hyper-connected homes. After all, phenomena of youth disengagement have been observed in different countries and labelled in various ways over the past few years. NEET ("Not in education, employment or training") is an acronym coined in the UK to describe young people who are not studying, not working and not even in job training.[34] *Slacker*, *twixter,* and *adultolescent* are terms used in the United States to describe young people who live with their parents and do not seek independence.[35] NEY ("Non-Engaged Youth") in Hong Kong refers to young people who do not have jobs and do not intend to continue their education.[36]

9.4 Some Final Questions

In conclusion, compared to the other forms of psychic distress and mental illness described in this book, hikikomori presents some peculiar characteristics. It has been said that it seems to be born at a precise moment within defined geographical and cultural coordinates, but it does not seem to be possible to guess when or within what boundaries its spread will end. Hikikomori could establish itself as the youth mental illness of the new century.

The resounding success of the hikikomori diagnosis, however, does not necessarily rule out the identification of different psychopathological conditions under the same name. Even the most recent literature reviews point out that there is still still no transnational project for "counting" cases of hikikomori. There are also no commonly accepted and rigorous criteria for a *differential diagnosis*, i.e. for distinguishing when a case is definable as hikikomori and when it is not. Such criteria should be included, for this purpose, in a future version of the DSM. There are no internationally used *diagnostic instruments*, such as structured interviews, i.e. standard lists of questions to be used by trained professionals, which are normally used for this purpose. Only uniformity of criteria, on the other hand, would allow psychiatrists and psychologists throughout the world to know whether they are using the word hikikomori to define truly comparable cases or only people who have certain symptoms in common. Keeping in mind that every mental illness, it can be said, has at least some symptoms in common with at least one other mental illness.

Thus, there is no certain way of establishing that one can diagnose hikikomori or *not*, for example, a personality disorder (schizotypal, schizoid, avoidant), a form of psychosis, or a form of depression. On the contrary, the possibility of identifying a *secondary* hikikomori makes a dual diagnosis *with* another disorder already defined by the DSM possible.

It may even be possible that in the near future this diagnostic category will be abandoned, and the symptoms will simply be considered new expressions of old disorders. It could be equally possible that the alleged spread of hikikomori outside Japan's borders is the result of an effort by Japanese psychiatrists to deny that the origin of the syndrome is to be identified solely in the peculiarities of their homeland's culture.[37] Equally possible, however, is that knowledge of the Japanese phenomenon abroad influenced its spread elsewhere, through a "patient to patient" communication, so to speak. If in Charcot's time, such communication could take place, perhaps, within the walls of the Salpêtrière, today there are virtually no walls that the Internet cannot cross.

Notes

1 Ricci, *Hikikomori: narrazioni da una porta chiusa*, 116.
2 Saito, *Hikikomori: Adolescence Without End*, 24.
3 Li and Wong, "Youth Social Withdrawal Behaviour".
4 Bagnato, *L'Hikikomori*.
5 Saito, *Hikikomori: Adolescence without End*, 32–33.
6 Koyama et al., "Lifetime Prevalence".
7 Heinze and Thomas, "Self and Salvation".
8 Watanabe, "Il mio mestiere di counseling e hikikomori".
9 Watanabe, "Il mio mestiere di counseling e hikikomori".
10 Bagnato, *L'hikikomori*.
11 Suwa and Suzuki, "The Phenomenon of Hikikomori".
12 Crepaldi, *Hikikomori: I giovani che non escono di casa*.
13 Crepaldi, *Hikikomori: I giovani che non escono di casa*.
14 Saito, "Preface".
15 Saito, *Hikikomori: Adolescence without End*.
16 Henshall, *Japanese Society*.
17 Zielenziger, *Shutting Out the Sun*.
18 Hiyama and Yoshihara, "New Occupational Threats".
19 Ricci and Piotti, *Hikikomori: adolescenti in volontaria reclusione*.
20 Saito, *Hikikomori: Adolescence without End*.
21 Ricci, *Hikikomori: narrazioni da una porta chiusa*.
22 Bagnato, *L'hikikomori*, 26.
23 Kato, Hashimoto et al., "Multidimensional Anatomy of Modern Type Depression".
24 Ricci, *Hikikomori: narrazioni da una porta chiusa*.
25 Kato, Shinfuku et al., "Loneliness and Single-person Households".
26 Li and Wong, "Youth Social Withdrawal Behaviour".
27 Kato, Shinfuku et al., "Are Japan's Hikikomori and Depression in Young People Spreading Abroad?".
28 Saito, "Preface".
29 Crepaldi, *Hikikomori: I giovani che non escono di casa*, 10.
30 Teo et al., "Identification of the Hikikomori Syndrome".
31 Malagón-Amor, et al., "Hikikomori in Spain".

32 Kato, Shinfuku et al., "Are Japan's Hikikomori and Depression in Young People Spreading Abroad?".
33 Saito, "Preface".
34 Bynner and Parsons, "Social Exclusion".
35 Staff, "Coming of Age in America".
36 Wong, "Social Withdrawal".
37 See, in particular, Saito, "Preface", compared to Saito, *Hikikomori: Adolescence Without End.*

10 The Misunderstanding of Homosexuality as a Form of Pathology

10.1 The Story of Alan

One morning in early March 1952, John Turing receives a letter from his brother Alan that begins with these words: "I suppose you know that I am a homosexual".[1] John, a respectable businessman in the City of London, knows nothing of the sort and immediately realises that the letter needs his full attention. He therefore decides to continue the letter to the office, folds it, and puts it in his breast pocket.

John knows a lot about his brother Alan Turing. He knows that he is considered a genius in his field. He knows that his work helped save the country during the Second World War. Although the matter is still classified as top secret, it is thanks to the prototype electronic calculator he built that it was possible to crack the German Enigma code and consequently know the contents of all the Third Reich's encrypted communications (the story was retold in the popular 2014 film *The Imitation Game*). John knows, or thinks he knows, that Alan is a misogynist. He has noticed how he avoids in the most absolute way flirting with girls in clubs in his presence. However, he would have never imagined to associate him to one of those "effeminate perverts" that constitute the category of homosexuals in his mind as a quiet bourgeois individual of the British Empire.

The letter, which John Turing finishes reading at his desk, explains the reason for that puzzling premise. In the United Kingdom of 1952, homosexuality is not only considered *abnormal* conduct but is even *illegal*. Another distinguished British citizen, Oscar Wilde, had suffered a trial for homosexuality a few decades earlier and had been sentenced to two years of hard labour. It was while in prison that Wilde wrote one of his most famous works, *De Profundis*, a kind of spiritual testament written in the form of an open letter to his unworthy and ungrateful partner Alfred Douglas.[2]

Alan Turing was arrested for homosexual conduct, on the basis of a five-page statement that he drafted and handed in to the police. Having suffered a burglary, Alan had reported it, omitting at first to specify that he knew the identity of the burglar very well, since he was having an affair with him. The thief, however, is known to the police, and is already

DOI: 10.4324/9781003481249-11

under arrest for other reasons and a comparison of fingerprints with those in Alan Turing's flat quickly revealed his identity. He was a 19-year-old named Arnold Murray, who had already been arrested for shoplifting in London and then released on parole. Alan had ended up admitting the nature of his relationship with Arnold, in the belief that the crime of homosexuality was considered venial and, on the way, out of the penal code. This was not the case. Laws punishing male homosexual conduct were repealed in England and Wales in 1967, in Scotland in 1980, in Northern Ireland in 1982. In the United States, a complete abolition of laws punishing homosexuality (both male and female, in this case) did not occur until 2003.[3]

The policemen interrogating Alan Turing pretend to be interested in the theft, but in fact the sexual misconduct of a member of the upper class intrigues them much more. The admissions in the written statement, which Alan naively thinks he is drafting in order to clarify the crime committed by Arnold Murray, actually incriminate himself. On 28 February, Alan Turing appeared before the judge for the first hearing and the circumstance appeared in the local newspapers, albeit, for the time being, without much prominence. Alan then wrote to his brother to prevent the news from reaching him sooner or later from other sources.

If fame had not saved Wilde, John Turing probably thinks, it would not have saved Alan either, whose brilliant insights and discoveries the world still knows little of. John therefore decides that his current affairs can be neglected for a couple of days and heads straight to Manchester, where his brother lives and faces trial on twelve counts, all relating to *gross indecency* with Arnold Murray. Alan's only, relative, good fortune is that he is not openly accused of *buggering* (sodomy), the penalty for which would be much more severe.

One thing above all worries John Turing. His brother's statement leaves no doubt about his conduct. Alan first met Arnold Murray in the street and, seeing him in a bad way, invited him for a bite to eat. Alan had found Arnold's appearance pleasing and enjoyed their conversation. He had therefore invited him to his home in the Wimslow area on several occasions and had been intimate with him, until the day he noticed that silver cutlery was missing from the house. All this was very clear and, when questioned by the cops as to why he felt confident enough to find in the other a willing person, Alan had quietly replied that a person in such precarious financial circumstances as Arnold could hardly afford to be choosy. Despite the fact that all this is already on record, Alan Turing has written to his brother that he intends to plead "not guilty", obviously in the belief that there is nothing in his conduct worthy of moral censure. John, in contrast to Alan, realises that such an attitude would be extremely dangerous. What Alan has quietly handed over to the cops is already enough to convict him. Only by pleading guilty can he secure a speedy trial, with as little publicity as possible and a relatively light sentence.

The Cambridge University environment proves to be very supportive. Alan informs Max Newman, his department head, of the incident in the middle of the cafeteria and in a loud voice, so as to leave no doubt that he feels he has nothing to hide. He will not be disappointed by what he sees as a kind of substitute father figure. Newman states unambiguously that it would be a severe mistake to deprive Alan of the post of *lecturer* and no higher academic authority intervenes to question his position. Not differently do the other friends react. Alan is then assured that, once left the prison, he will be able to continue working.

The trial, however, saw him convicted, with an alternative choice between two years in prison and chemical castration. In those very years, treatments with oestrogens were being tested, to be administered to homosexuals, which were supposed to cancel libido completely for the time of administration. Theoretically, at the end of the oestrogen administration period, one should return to the previous condition, but the side effects on psyche and soma are still not perfectly clear and Alan Turing ends up turning into an impotent guinea pig. In addition to losing his desire, he begins to develop mild gynaecomastia (breast growth) and goes into depression. He is found dead by his maid on 8 June 1954. An autopsy reveals traces of potassium cyanide in his body: death by poisoning is quickly dismissed as suicide. It was not until 2013 that Queen Elizabeth II signed a posthumous pardon for Turing, following a campaign by several famous scientists (including Stephen Hawking) to mark the centenary of his birth.

10.2 The Paradox of the Norm

Homosexuality, the subject of this chapter, is not a form of psychopathology with peculiar historical-geographical characteristics; actually, it is simply not a form of psychopathology. Rather, it can be defined as a sexual orientation that, although not in the majority, cannot today be considered pathological, even if for long historical periods has been considered as such, in a non-univocal way. In the course of the following pages, it will be made clear why it is particularly difficult to use "normality" as a benchmark here. In some cases, homosexuals reclaim the possibility of being considered "normal", in others the pride of considering themselves "different".

We anticipate that, for the time being, we will refer to homosexuality as sexual desire for and sexual practice with persons of one's own sex, and will dispense with any consideration of the more articulated expressions of gender identity and sexuality, now summarised in the acronym LGBTQIA+.

In today's world, to think that a few decades ago in a Western nation homosexual orientation could be criminally sanctioned may seem puzzling, but in the Catholic cultural context, the stigma towards homosexuality is still present. In that environment, homosexual relations are in fact still often defined as "against nature", despite the fact that in nature homosexual conduct affects numerous species, both in captivity and in the wild.

As Vittorio Lingiardi reports, the term "homosexual" was invented in 1869 by the Hungarian writer Károly Mária Kertheny (1824–1882), who used it in an anonymous pamphlet against the introduction by the Prussian Ministry of Justice of a law punishing sexual acts between male persons.[4] Paradoxically, then, it is possible that the identification of homosexuality as a form of psychopathology, in this case perversion, constituted a kind of progress in the 19th century:

> Homosexuality was then a vice, and homosexual practices were condemned and produced a very consistent feeling of guilt in homosexuals. According to Krafft-Ebing, however, the homosexual is not an immoral or bad man, but a man who suffers from a perversion of the normal instincts. The homosexual is a pervert and a pervert is a sick person. This classification seems oppressive and feels like a condemnation, but at the time doctors considered it a liberation from moral stigmata.[5]

In any case, homosexuality is probably the only form of alleged psychopathology that, at least for a time, was considered a crime in itself, although not the only one for which imprisonment was provided. Understandably, however, detention in prison is different from detention in a mental health institution. It should be noted that the word "treatment" was in many cases a term used euphemistically. Alan Turing, who was considered one of the scientific geniuses of the 20th century and a decisive architect of the Allied military advantage during the Second World War, died as a result of the fact that British laws considered homosexuality a crime, no more than seventy years ago. On the other hand, the claim of normality of homosexual conduct has led to civil battles for the recognition of rights of same-sex couples, including the possibility of marriage and adoption.[6] Finally, there is no shortage of those who have challenged the very idea of normative rules in this sphere, observing that the institution of same-sex marriage would delegitimise those possibilities of kinship, familiarity, and cohabitation that transcend the principle of the couple as the basis of the family and society:

> No doubt, marriage and same-sex domestic partnerships should certainly be available as options, but to install either as a model for sexual legitimacy is precisely to constrain the sociality of the body in acceptable ways.[7]

In other words, there are those who regard homosexuality as abnormal in a pejorative sense, those who claim their normality, and those who claim their radical diversity. Judith Butler, discussing the Vatican's firm opposition in the United Nations to considering homosexuals' rights as human rights, writes:

> It is for me no surprise that the Vatican refers to the possible inclusion of lesbian rights as 'anti-human'. Perhaps that is true. To admit the lesbian into the realm of the universal might be to undo the human, at least in its present form, but it might also be to imagine the human beyond its conventional limits.[8]

The attitude towards homosexuality on the part of Western culture has varied widely throughout history: acceptance, tolerance, condemnation are the three prevailing terms with which this attitude can be described from time to time. Condemnation on the part of the heterosexual majority has for many centuries been fairly unequivocal in Europe and the United States. At times there were moments characterised by tolerance, i.e. the idea that the homosexual was on the one hand a deviant from "natural" conduct, and on the other hand should not be punished, stigmatised, or even cured for it. Acceptance, i.e. the possibility of considering homosexuality as a "normal" variant of human sexuality, may be considered a conquest, or rather a re-conquest, of the late 20th century, but it is nevertheless by far the prevailing attitude within the psychiatric and psychotherapeutic community today.

One can speak of re-conquest because in classical antiquity the picture was different from what one might expect. In ancient Greece, homosexual eros was considered the most authentic form of love, at least that between men.

> Greek culture differed from ours in its readiness to recognise the alternation of homosexual and heterosexual preferences in the same individual, its implicit denial that such alternation or coexistence created peculiar problems for the individual or for society, its sympathetic response to the open expression of homosexual desire in words and behaviour, and its taste for the uninhibited treatment of homosexual subjects in literature and the visual arts.[9]

In particular, it was considered natural for the young *ephebe*, still immature, to receive the attentions of a more experienced man, in a relationship that was technically called an *orthòs paiderasthéin*, literally "a correct form of pederasty". *Orthòs paiderasthéin* was not merely tolerated, but sometimes actively promoted, as for instance in 5th century Athens.[10] Nor did this kind of relationship invalidate in the eyes of others the masculinity of the two involved, even with respect to warlike virtues. Achilles, in the *Iliad*, is the ephebe of Patroclus.[11] At Thebes, an elite unit of the army, known as the "Sacred Band of Thebes", lined up side by side select soldiers who had sexual relations with each other, according to the principle that the bond "cemented by friendship grounded upon love is never to be broken, and invincible; since the lovers ashamed to be base in sight of their beloved, and the beloved before their lovers, willingly rush into danger for the relief of one another. that exists between beings who love each other is indissoluble and unbreakable. There the lovers for shame of the beloved, and these for shame of the lovers will resist in dangers, defending each other".[12]

What, if anything, constituted the discriminating factor between socially approved and disapproved behaviour was the age of the beloved. Once the age of development was over and the secondary sexual characteristics were fully visible, the passive role had to be definitively abandoned in favour of the active one. Remaining out of the passive role was stigmatised, just as the Oriental (Persian in particular) habit of shaving one's beard was considered a sign of effeminacy and decadence. It can be seen, therefore, that albeit in different forms, the tendency to "normalise" sexuality is present in this historical era as it will be in subsequent ones.

The two main treatises on love in Greek antiquity speak of male homosexual eros and compare it to heterosexual eros. Plato's *Symposium* argues for the existence of two kinds of eros and two goddesses of love: a celestial Aphrodite and a vulgar one, to whom the less noble eros pertains. In this regard, the character Pausanias says, not contradicted by any of the participants in the dialogue: "Now the Love that belongs to the Popular Aphrodite is in very truth popular and does his work at haphazard: this is the Love we see in the meaner sort of men: who, in the first place, love women as well as boys; secondly, where they love, they are set on the body more than the soul".[13] Here it is clear that it is heterosexual love that is considered less noble. Socrates, at the end of the *Symposium*, is extolled by the beautiful Alcibiades, as the object of homosexual desire.

The perspective changes slightly in Plutarch's *Dialogue in Love*, where the story of the ephebe Bacchon and the rich and attractive widow Ismedonora who wants to marry him serves as a backdrop for general considerations on love. The interlocutors are scandalised because they will be deprived of the possibility of enjoying Bacchon's graces as a result of his marriage to a woman. Yet they are told that, after all, a woman has the right to love a man as well as another man. The Platonic conception is corrected, but not overturned: "'But,' you may say, 'there is much that is bas and mad in the love of women.' And doesn't that of boys have even more?".[14]

It has been pointed out above that the homosexual eros that was accepted and indeed celebrated by the Greeks was essentially male. Much less can be said about female homoerotic eros, basically because classical Greece is a world of men described by men. However, one cannot forget that homoerotic love is sung by Sappho, the greatest Greek poetess and undoubtedly one of the greatest poets of all time:

> Love bittersweet, irrepressible, loosens my limbs and I tremble. Yet, Atthis, you despise my being. To chase Andromeda you leave me. Once more Love stirs me up, the limb-loosener, a creature bitter-sweet, baffling.[15]

After all, two of the most commonly used adjectives to designate female homosexuality are "sapphic", from Sappho's name, and "lesbian", from the island of Lesbos, where she was born.

In the world of ancient Rome, for a long time the attitude towards sexuality was not very different from that of classical Greece:

> For the Greeks and Romans, the fundamental bipartition between sexual behaviour was not between hetero- and homo-sexuality, but rather between activity and passivity. For them, virility meant and imposed 'activity'. A man was expected to be active in all fields, from war, in which he had to win, to politics, in which he had to impose his ideas, to love, in which he had to subdue not only women, but also some men.[16]

This is why the passive role was, in general, until the late Republican era delegated to slaves and considered unworthy of a free man. The fact that Cicero, in one of the *Philippicae*, alludes with contempt to the relationship of Mark Antony and Curion, which was in the public domain, signals the fact that times were changing in that regard. In the imperial age, it is even possible that gay marriages were legalised. In any case, several sources (including Tacitus and Suetonius) attest that Nero was the protagonist on at least two occasions of official marriage ceremonies with other men, both as "groom" and "bride".[17]

The acceptance of homosexuality as guilt-free conduct not deserving of condemnation ceases with the establishment of Christianity, which inherited the Old Testament attitude to sexual morality. Homosexual conduct is defined as an *abomination* in *Leviticus*, alongside prostitution, adultery, and even sexual intercourse during the menstrual cycle, for which capital punishment is evoked. The inclusion of homosexual intercourse among *impure acts* (contrary to the sixth commandment) is clear and – despite some recent interpretations – there does not seem to be any explicit correction in the Gospels. The condemnation of homosexuality is rather unequivocal by various Church fathers and seems unquestionable in the two best-known voices in the history of Christian theology, those of Augustine of Hippo and Thomas Aquinas.[18]

The designation "sin" has not in itself merited civil and moral sanction in Christian society. Hypocrites and gluttons are sinners in the same way as homosexuals, according to Holy Scripture, yet neither the former nor the latter have ever been persecuted. On the contrary, in the course of time, there have been legislations condemning gays to the stake and explicitly authorising prostitution, even though it also implied *an impure act*.[19] However, it should not be assumed that such a level of execration and condemnation characterised homosexuality in the eyes of Christian culture from the very beginning. Several centuries passed from the abolition of homosexual marriages, dating back to the 4th century,[20] to the affirmation of the Counter-Reformation idea of the homosexual as a *danger* to society, in the same way as witches and usurers (the latter were particularly execrated especially because they were necessarily identified with Jews, the only ones authorised to lend money at interest).[21] The sin of homosexuality, in fact, was tolerated like many others up to the threshold of the late Middle Ages. For example, the same 18th-century manual for confessors that condemned *impure acts* between men to one year's penance ("only" one hundred and sixty days were sufficient for impure acts between women) suggested that three years' penance be imposed on a priest who went hunting.[22] Even in the 14th century, in Dante's *Commedia* it is noted that, although sodomites are condemned in no small way, one of them, Brunetto Latini, is one of the figures Dante looks upon most sympathetically in the first canticle.[23]

In any case, from the Counter-Reformation to the 19th century, in the Western European world homosexuality was considered abnormal, dangerous, and deserving of condemnation in an almost unequivocal manner. Paradoxically, it is precisely its identification as a "mental illness" that lays the foundations for a change, because the sick person as such cannot be considered guilty of their own infirmity. As a form of psychopathology, however, homosexuality remained beyond the wall of what is considered normal and acceptable. The wall slowly began to be breached by Freud's psychoanalysis, who took up from his friend and confidant Wilhelm Fliess the idea that the human being is by nature bisexual. Freud, for example, writes in a note in *Civilisation and Its Discontents*:

> Man is an animal organism with (like others) an unmistakably bisexual disposition. The individual corresponds to a fusion of two symmetrical halves, of which, according to some investigators, one is purely male and the other female. It is equally possible that each half was originally hermaphrodite. Sex is a biological fact which, although it is of extraordinary importance in mental life, is hard to grasp psychologically.[24]

Homosexual "object choice" would therefore be potentially present from the beginning for all human beings. Freud, however, saw it in fact as a deviation from normal adult genital sexuality carried out following a fixation on the mother figure and an identification with her, the result of which would be the choice of love objects similar to oneself. A choice therefore made, according to Freud, "on the path of narcissism". In Jung's view, one can also speak of a kind of psychological bisexuality of the human being. Every man would be characterised by a female unconscious component (the *anima*) and every woman by a male unconscious component (the *animus*). Homosexuality would simply consist of an identification with the counter-sexual components of oneself. Georg Groddeck, a heterodox analyst to whom Freud was very close, went so far as to write: "Yes, I hold the view that all people are homosexual, hold it so firmly that it is difficult for me to realise how anyone can think differently".[25]

Despite these standpoints, the history of psychoanalysis has certainly not coincided with fighting prejudice against homosexuals. This became clear, for example, when the psychoanalytic movement found itself debating whether to admit homosexuals to training as future analysts. As is well known, the first two training institutes were founded in Vienna and Berlin:

> While the Viennese, under the leadership of Otto Rank, had called for assessing each case on its own individual merits, the majority of the Berliners, led by Karl Abraham, insisted that if psychoanalysis had not cured an individual of his or her 'inversion', then he or she was also incapable of being an analyst.[26]

In the United Kingdom, Ernest Jones, despite Freud's open dissent, actively advocated the rejection of homosexuals as analyst candidates in 1921 and most British analysts shared the same view.[27] The only exception was Edward Glover who, despite classifying homosexuality as a form of perversion ("the most advanced and organised"), argued that "the manifestations of homosexual love-feeling and the attitude to the love object cannot be distinguished from those associated with normal heterosexual love".[28] Glover was also the only analyst in England to officially take a stand for the decriminalisation of homosexuality.[29]

In short, despite Freud, prejudice towards homosexuality prevailed among psychoanalysts for a long time,[30] especially when psychoanalysis, in order to establish itself, largely had to identify with dominant ideologies and prejudices.[31] The first decisive push towards overcoming the idea of homosexuality as a psychopathology came from the world of sexology. The so-called "Kinsey Reports", which were widely circulated, revealed how large a percentage of people practised homosexual conduct.[32] In fact, the work of the sexologist Alfred Kinsey represented a very strong *endorsement*, from a scientific point of view, for a greater "democratic pluralism of sexuality", as it was expressed at the time.[33] In 1957, an experiment by Evelyn Hooker demonstrated that "there are no psychopathological markers of homosexuality [...] and therefore homosexuality cannot be considered a diagnostic category".[34]

In 1973, the American Psychiatric Association (APA) decided to distinguish between ego-syntonic and ego-dystonic homosexuality, i.e. between serene acceptance or discomfort with one's homosexual inclinations. In the subsequent reissue of the DSM,[35] only the ego-dystonic version was included. In a specific panel at the APA congress held in May of that year, three psychiatrists in particular argued for the historic change: Robert Stoller, Judd Marmor, and Richard Green. Stoller, who had published the seminal *Sex and Gender* in 1968, was the only psychoanalyst of the trio, but he was particularly effective in arguing how different variants of heterosexual conduct – sexual promiscuity, preference for prostitutes, use of pornography, adult masturbation – deserved, at best, more clinical attention than homosexuality as such. From this point of view, Nancy Chodorow's 1992 paramount essay, entitled *Heterosexuality as a Compromise Formation*, would complete the reversal of perspective. According to Chodorow, it is only the fact that heterosexuality is culturally taken for granted that prevents one from seeing how it can constitute a landing place devoid of psychopathological problems in itself.[36]

In 1990, even ego-dystonic homosexuality was deleted from possible diagnoses in DSM-IV[37], and the same happened in 1993 with the ICD-10, published by the WHO.[38] From that moment on, for mental health professionals, one can no longer speak of pathology related to homosexuality, nor of a possible "cure", except in the sense of helping the ego-dystonic homosexual to accept his or her tendencies. Dystonia is in fact generally interpreted as a product of the culture of reference. The Catholic milieu, for example, has continued to consider homosexuality a mental disorder and a sin and to promote so-called "reparative therapies", aimed at changing a sexual orientation considered to be against nature. If, however, Catholic psychiatrists have continued to speak of a "controversial homosexual issue",[39] other mental health professionals have now taken a unanimous position. There is a specific statement by the APA against reparative therapies, published in 2000.[40]

Today, we may be surprised by the fact that homosexuality could have been considered a form of pathology until so recently. Perhaps we should not forget how facts that today seem to have been acquired are the result of recent cultural conquests, such as women's right to vote, the right to divorce, the right to abortion. We should not forget how prejudice against a skin colour other than one's own has not abandoned large strata of the population. And we should not forget that what has been learnt is not necessarily learnt once and for all. Homosexuality continues to be stigmatised even in the West in various homophobic contexts. Homophobia, once considered "normal", is now viewed with suspicion by mental health professionals.

Notes

1 Hodges, *Alan Turing: The Enigma*, 322.
2 Wilde, *De Profundis*.
3 Nussbaum, "Preface".
4 Lingiardi, *Citizen Gay*, 31.
5 Hacking, *Façonner les gens*, 41.
6 An overview of the recent history of these battles can be found in Lingiardi, *Citizan Gay*.
7 Butler, *Undoing Gender*, 26.
8 Butler, *Undoing Gender*, 190.
9 Dover, *Greek Homosexuality*, 30.
10 Halperin, *One Hundred Years of Homosexuality*.
11 Plato, *Symposium* (180a), 180–181.
12 Plutarch, *Life of Pelopidas* (17), 357.
13 Plato, *Symposium* (181°–b), 108–109.
14 Plutarch, *Dialogue on Love* (769b), 426–427.

15 Sappho, *Lyrics* (130), 24–25.
16 Cantarella, *Secondo natura*, 10.
17 Williams, *Roman Homosexuality*, 279.
18 Augustine of Hippo, *Confessions*, 3; Thomas Aquinas, *Summa Theologica*, ii–ii (q 154, a 12).
19 Boswell, *Christianity, Social Tolerance, and Homosexuality.*
20 Williams, *Roman Homosexuality.*
21 Taradel, *L'accusa del Sangue.*
22 Boswell, *Christianity, Social Tolerance, and Homosexuality.*
23 Dante Alighieri, *Inferno*, XV.
24 Freud, *Civilisation and Its Discontents*, 104, note 3.
25 Groddeck, *The Book of the Id*, 199.
26 Herzog, *Cold War Freud*, 61.
27 Lingiardi, *Citizen Gay.*
28 Glover, *Psycho-analysis*, 257.
29 Glover, *The Roots of Crime.*
30 Lingiardi, *Citizen Gay.*
31 Herzog, *Cold War Freud.*
32 Kinsey, Pomeroy, Martin, and Gebhard, *Sexual Behaviour in the Human Male*; Kinsey, Pomeroy, Martin, and Gebhard, *Sexual Behaviour in the Human Female.*
33 Herzog, *Cold War Freud.*
34 Lingiardi, *Citizen Gay*, 95.
35 APA, *DSM-II.*
36 Chodorow, "Heterosexuality as a Compromise Formation".
37 APA, *DSM-IV.*
38 World Health Organisation, *The ICD-10 Classification of Mental and Behavioural Disorders.*
39 Cantelmi, *Cattolici e Psiche.*
40 APA, "Official Statement of the APA on Attempts to Change Sexual Orientation".

Some Brief Final Considerations

It should have been sufficiently illustrated how each cultural context can, on the one hand, give rise to specific forms of distress, which in our language we can call forms of psychopathology; on the other hand, label as pathological something that in itself would not be so; finally, determine a stigmatisation towards diversity. By contrast, the suffering that follows is very often genuine.

In the last chapter, we saw a dramatic example of how sexuality other than that which the majority perceives as "normal" has historically been stigmatised as vicious, sinful, or perverse. If, however, what is characteristic of a portion of humanity (in this case, homosexuals) can be classified as "abnormal" for centuries, it is easy to imagine the risk of labelling and marginalisation that the individual who does not conform to the demands of his or her own culture can run.

One can here propose a paradoxical example of a multiple "diagnosis" applied to a character who fortunately was immune to risk and is generally considered today one of psychology's creative geniuses: Carl Gustav Jung. When Jung broke away from the psychoanalytic movement in 1913, Freud and his students went to great lengths to describe him as mentally ill. If Freud's and Eissler's positions were politically motivated and can be historically contextualised,[1] much less understandable is such a position on the part of authors of Jung biographies who as such could have studied works and archival documents accurately. Yet it will be found that Paul Stern described him as a semi-psychotic visionary;[2] Vincent Brome as a manic-depressive personality;[3] Gerhard Wehr as a case on the borderline between neurosis and psychosis;[4] Frank McLynn more generically as suffering from an unspecified mental illness;[5] Deirdre Bair as subject to psychotic visions.[6] One can therefore understand that, in the wrong context, a poor *dropout* who does not enjoy the prestige and social status of someone like Jung can run very serious risks.[7]

The attempt to draw up a form of classification of mental illness with an a-theoretical character, i.e. independent of any theory, is necessarily doomed to failure, because, as it has been pointed out in the course of the preceding pages, there is no objective way to consider observational data. Whenever we

DOI: 10.4324/9781003481249-12

observe something, we depend on assumptions.[8] The case of the DSM is particularly significant in this respect. Despite being created with the intention of providing a common instrument for psychiatrists and clinical psychologists of different tendencies, without privileging any of them, it ended up promoting a kind of potential psychiatry of any kind of conduct.

Only one example will be given here: *Tobacco Use Disorder*, which is a specific diagnosis in the DSM-5.[9] The definition of "a significant pattern of tobacco use that leads to discomfort" could apply to many smokers, such as "tobacco is often taken in larger quantities or over a longer period than intended" (criterion 1) and "in situations in which it is physically dangerous (e.g. smoking in bed)" (criterion 8). Given that satisfying two of the numerous criteria is sufficient, once "distress" has been established, one can understand how easy it is to apply such a diagnosis, which is to all intents and purposes a psychiatric diagnosis. Acknowledging the risks of indiscriminate pathologisation, the Chair of the task force that drafted the DSM-IV, Allen Frances, after seeing the DSM-5 published, published a book entitled *Saving Normal: An Insider's Revolt Against Out-of-Control Psychiatric Diagnosis.*[10]

Furthermore, there are cases in which an apparently broad consensus on the definition of a psychopathology is not matched by a similar unanimity in its practical application. Schizophrenia is probably one of these cases, if one agrees that there are such ambiguous cases "for which the diagnosis of schizophrenia sheds less light on the patient than on the psychiatrist's choice on which the diagnosis is based".[11] Another elusive diagnosis is that of "Borderline Personality Disorder" (BPD). Although this disorder has had its own apparently clear definition in the DSM for a long time, in fact: (1) many patients can also be diagnosed as having different personality disorders (e.g. "Histrionic Personality Disorder"); (2) some researchers, such as Drew Westen, argue that such a disorder, as it is described in the DSM, in fact does not exist in nature;[12] (3) several psychiatrists employ the diagnosis of borderline as a kind of "bin" where they throw all cases in which they do not feel sure what to write in the medical record; (4) some analysts, such as Kernberg,[13] use the word "borderline" both in the specific meaning of the DSM[14] and in a broader sense, in which they basically encompass all personality disorders (the PDM has also followed a similar approach)[15]. Moreover, the entire Lacanian world refuses to consider such a category sensible, identifying a part of the cases diagnosed by others as "borderline" as psychotic and the remaining part as hysterical.

Expectations as to the desired result can also be a prerequisite not without risk. We have seen how the Hippocratic followers were looking for a drug that would expel black bile and believed they found it in a poison that caused the expulsion of digested blood.[16] In the mid-20th century, psychiatrists seeking to obtain less agitated behaviour from some psychotics believed they could achieve this through prefrontal lobotomy, only to discover that the price to be paid was the integrity of the patients' minds.[17] The development of psychopharmacology has certainly improved the lives of many people, but the abuse of psychotropic drugs has had far less positive results.

The attempt to mythologise madness as a form of creativity, which has characterised the most extreme forms of anti-psychiatric experiences, can certainly be risky. In Italy, there was a period during which, following the closure of asylums with the "Law 180",[18] madness was considered in certain circles a mark of creativity and emancipation from the repressed bourgeois world. On the other hand, even the misuse of compulsory health treatments is by no means risk-free. In Italy, the TSO ("trattamento sanitario obbligatorio", i.e. "compulsory mental health hospitalisation") in fact provides not only for the detention, albeit temporary, of the person subjected to it, but also the possibility of his or her restraint, with outcomes that can be in some cases inauspicious, or even fatal.[19]

In the field of mental health as in any other field, therefore, legitimate and desirable trust in scientific knowledge must always go hand in hand with an awareness of its possible limitations and provisionality.

We can close this book with a brief consideration of the epistemological consequences that can be drawn from the observation of the connection of mental illness with both culture and nature. The contrast between realism and constructivism was recalled in the introduction. Freud, who adhered strictly to scientific realism, was also a reductionist. In fact, he expressed his belief in both psychic determinism (every mental phenomenon has a series of precise mental causes) and physical determinism (every phenomenon has specific physical causes). Even with this position, however, Freud also claimed the reality of mental phenomena, which are certainly not illusory. He was nevertheless convinced that it was possible to describe universal laws of the psyche and presented the psychoanalytic theory as valid regardless of historical-geographical coordinates.

His successors, on the other hand, have abundantly demonstrated how Freud's is only *one* of the possible points of view with respect to a *specific* culture. However, even the pure constructivist perspective, proves unacceptable in the face of the realisation that, despite their diversity, various mental illnesses linked to different cultural contexts may have common elements that are evidently traceable to brain phenomena. A mental illness can certainly be simulated (by those who suffer from it or by those who describe it, as in the case of sluggish schizophrenia), but even in this borderline case, the phenomenon has its own level of reality, because the psychological consequences of the simulation on one's own or others' mind are in any case an observable phenomenon. In most cases, however, mental illness can be interpreted (like individual personality, for that matter) as the product of several factors: subjective experience, inter-subjective experience (dual, familial, group, popular, historical), and material factors (physical, chemical, neuro-physiological).

The phenomenology of mental illness constitutes one of the evident demonstrations that "the mind has causal powers that are neither reducible to the laws investigated by the natural sciences nor incompatible with them".[20] This does not mean adhering to the "party of the soul" as Douglas Hofstadter called it,[21] but to a perspective that has been called "quasi-naturalism" or "liberalised naturalism", which "although consistent with the laws of nature, is neither guided nor purely derived" from physics and medicine.[22]

Notes

1 Freud, *On the History of the Psychoanalytic Movement*; Eissler, *Psychological Aspects of the Correspondence Between Freud and Jung.*
2 Stern, *C. G. Jung: The Haunted Prophet.*
3 Brome, *Jung: Man and Myth.*
4 Wehr, *Jung: A Biography.*
5 McLynn, *Carl Gustav Jung.*
6 Bair, *Jung: A Biography.* An extensive discussion of the numerous flaws in most of Jung's biographies can be found in Shamdasani, *Jung Stripped Bare.*
7 Foschi (ed.), *La libertà sospesa.*
8 Hanson, *Patterns of Discovery.*
9 American Psychiatric Association, *DSM-5*, 666–667.
10 Frances, *Saving Normal.* In *DSM-5-TR* the Tobacco Use disorder needs only two criteria in order to be diagnosed. Among the criteria, for example: "Tobacco is often taken in larger amounts [...] than was intended" (criterion 1); "[...] a strong desire [...] to use tobacco" (3); "Recurrent tobacco use in situations in which it is physically hazardous (e.g., smoking in bed" (8) (American Psychiatric Association, *DSM-5-TR*, 645).
11 Blankenburg, *Der Verlust der natürlichen Selbstverständlichkeit*, 63.
12 Westen, Shedler, and Lingiardi, *La valutazione della personalità.*
13 Kernberg, *Severe Personality Disorders*; Kernberg and Caligor, "A Psychoanalytic Theory of Personality Disorders".
14 American Psychiatric Association, *DSM-5-TR.*
15 Lingiardi and McWilliams, *Psychodynamic Diagnostic Manual PDM-2.*
16 Onians, *The Origins of European Thought.*
17 Foschi and Innamorati, *A Critical History of Psychotherapy.*
18 The "Law 180" is more famously known as "Legge Basaglia", taking its name from its main proponent, the Italian psychiatrist Franco Basaglia. It was a revolutionary mental health act (1978) which substantially reformed the psychiatric system in Italy, by leading to the closing down of all psychiatric hospitals and their gradual replacement with a wide range of community-based services and settings for acute in-patient care.
19 Foschi, *La libertà sospesa.*
20 De Caro, *Realtà*, 84.
21 Hofstadter, *Gödel, Escher, Bach.*
22 Rudder Baker, *Naturalism*, 233.

Bibliography

Alcindor, Louis, and Maurat, Paul. "Un cas d'hystérie avec automatisme ambulatoire et tremblement". *Gazette des Hôpitaux* 8 (1889): 253–254.
Amorth, Gabriele. *Esorcisti e psichiatri*. Bologna: Edb, 2000.
American Psychiatric Association. *DSM-II. Diagnostic and Statistical Manual of Mental Disorders*. Washington, DC: American Psychiatric Association, 1974.
American Psychiatric Association. *DSM-III-R. Diagnostic and Statistical Manual of Mental Disorders*. Washington, DC: American Psychiatric Association, 1987.
American Psychiatric Association. *DSM-III. Diagnostic and Statistical Manual of Mental Disorders*. Washington, DC: American Psychiatric Association, 1908.
American Psychiatric Association. *DSM-IV-TR. Diagnostic and Statistical Manual of Mental Disorders, Text Revision*. Washington, DC: American Psychiatric Association, 2000.
American Psychiatric Association. *DSM-IV. Diagnostic and Statistical Manual of Mental Disorders*. Washington, DC: American Psychiatric Association, 1994.
American Psychiatric Association. *DSM-5-TR. Diagnostic and Statistical Manual of Mental Disorders*. Washington, DC: American Psychiatric Association, 2022.
American Psychiatric Association. *DSM-5. Diagnostic and Statistical Manual of Mental Disorders*. Washington, DC: American Psychiatric Association, 2013.
American Psychiatric Association. "Official Statement of the American Psychiatric Association on Attempts to Change Sexual Orientation (Reparative or Conversion therapies)". *The American Journal of Psychiatry* 157/10 (2000): 1719–1721.
Aragon, Louis, and Breton, André. "Le cinquantenaire de l'hystérie (1878–1928)". *La révolution surréaliste* 11 (1928): 20–22.
Augustine of Hippo. *Confessions*. Edited by Henry Chadwick. Oxford: Oxford University Press, 2008.
Azam, Eugène. *Hypnotisme, double conscience et altérations de la personnalité*. Paris: G. Baillière, 1887.
Baglivi, Giorgio. "De anatome morsu et effectibus tarantulae". *Opera Omnia Medico-practica, Et Anatomica*. Bloomington, IL: Arkose Press, 2015. [Original work issued 1695]
Bagnato, Karin. *L'hikikomori: un fenomeno di autoreclusione giovanile*. Rome: Carocci, 2017.
Bair, Deirdre. *Jung: A Biography*. New York: Little Brown, 2003.
Balducci, Corrado. "Criterio diagnostico della possessione diabolica". In *La sfida di Belzebuul. Complessità psichica e possessione diabolica*, edited by Eugenio Fizzotti, 69–80. Rome: LAS, 1995.
Balducci, Corrado. *Il diavolo*. Milan: Mondadori, 1994.
Ballard, E. F. "Letters, Notes, and Answers". *British Medical Journal* 1/2672 (1912): 652 [https://www.bmj.com/content/1/2672/651]

Barbavara, G. "Esorcismo". In *Lexicon (Lessico Ecclesiastico Illustrato)*, vol. 2, 227. Milan: Vallardi, 1902.

Bayle, Antoine Laurent Jessé. *Traité des maladies du cerveau et de ses membranes*. Paris: Gabon, 1826.

Beaune, Jean Claude. *Le vagabond et la machine: essai sur l'automatisme ambulatoire: médicine, technique et société en France 1880–1910)*. Paris: Editions Champ Vallon, 1983.

Behr, Felix, L. Croq, and C. Vauterin, "Sémiologie des conduites de fugues". *Encyclopedie Medico-Chirurgicale. Psychiatrie* 37/113 A 10 (1985), 685–696.

Beneduce, Roberto. *Trance e possessione in Africa*. Turin: Bollati Boringhieri, 2002.

Berrios, German. *History of the Mental Symptoms*. New York: Cambridge University Press, 1996.

Bertrando, Paolo, and Toffanetti, Dario. *Storia della terapia familiare*. Milan: Raffaello Cortina, 2000.

Bird, Isabella L. *The Golden Chersonese and the Way Thither*. London: John Murray, 1883.

Blankenburg, Wolfganf. *Der Verlust der natürlichen Selbstverständlichkeit*. Berlin: Parodos Verlag, 1971.

Bleuler, Eugen. *Dementia Praecox or the Group of Schizophrenias*, edited by Joseph Zinker. New York: International Universities Press 1950. [Original work issued 1911].

Boas, Franz. "The Religion of the Kawkiutl". *Columbia University Contributions in Anthropology* 10/2 (1930): 1–41.

Boddy, Janice. "Spirit Possession Revisited: Beyond Instrumentality". *Annual Review of Anthropology* 23/1 (1994): 407–434.

Bogoras, Waldemar. "Chukchee Mythology. Jesup North Pacific Expedition". In *Memoirs of the American Museum of Natural History*, vol. 12. Leiden-New York: Brill and Stechert, 1910.

Bogoras, Waldemar. "The Chukchee Religion. Jesup North Pacific Expedition". In *Memoirs of the American Museum of Natural History*, vol. 7. Leiden-New York: Brill and Stechert, 1907.

Boindala, Naavena Sasikeran, Phebe Tucker, and Richard P. Trautman. "Culture and Psychiatry: A Course for Second-Year Psychiatry Residents". *Academic Psychiatry*, 37/1 (2013): 46–50.

Boswell, John. *Christianity, Social Tolerance, and Homosexuality: Gay People in Western Europe from the Beginning of the Christian Era to the Fourteenth Century*. Chicago: University of Chicago Press, 1908.

Breuer, Josef, and Freud, Sigmund, "Studies on Hysteria". In *The Standard Edition of the Complete Psychological Works of Sigmund Freud*, edited by James Strachey, vol. 2. London: Hogarth Press, 1955. [Original work issued 1895]

Bromberg, Philip M. *Awakening the Dreamer: Clinical Journeys*. London: Routledge, 2010.

Bromberg, Philip M. *Standing in the Spaces: Essays on Clinical Process Trauma and Dissociation*. London: Routledge, 2001.

Bromberg, Philip M. *The Shadow of the Tsunami. The Growth of the Relational Mind*. London: Routledge, 2011.

Brome, Vincent. *Jung: Man and Myth*. London: MacMillan, 1978.

Buber, Martin. *Die Schriften über das dialogische Prinzip*. Heidelberg: Lambert Schneider, 1954.

Burgl, Georg. "Eine Reise in die Schweiz im epileptischen Dämmerzustande und die transitorischen Bewusstseinsstörungen der Epileptiker vor dem Strafrichter". *Münchener medizinische Wochenschrift* 37 (1900): 1270–1273.

Butler, Judith. *Undoing Gender*. London: Routledge, 2004.

Bynner, John, and Parsons, Samantha. "Social Exclusion and the Transition from School to Work: The Case of Young People not in Education, Employment or Training". *Journal of Vocational Behaviour* 60 (2002): 289–309.

Call, Josep, and Tomasello, Michael. Eds. *The Gestural Communication of Apes and Monkeys*. Hove: Psychology Press, 2007.

Cantarella, Eva. *Secondo natura. La bisessualità nel mondo antico*. Milan: Feltrinelli, 2016.

Cantelmi, Tonino. *Cattolici e psiche. La controversa questione omosessuale*. Rome: San Paolo, 2008.

Cantelmi, Tonino, Pasquale Laselva, and Silvestro Paluzzi. *Psicologia e teologia in dialogo*. Rome: San Paolo, 2004.

Capizzi, Antonio. *L'uomo a due anime* [The Man with Two Souls]. Florence: La Nuova Italia, 1988.

Cartwright, Samuel Adolphus. "Report on the Diseases and Physical Peculiarities of the Negro Race". In *Concepts of Health and Disease: Interdisciplinary Perspectives*, edited by Arthur L. Caplan, Hugo Tristan Engelhardt Jr., and James J. McCartney, 305–326. Reading MA: Addison-Wesley, 1851.

Cazzato, Mario. "La taranta filologa: un medico (R. Mead), la fortuna di Baglivi in Inghilterra, la 'sfortuna' di Epifanio Ferdinando e dei 'sanpaolari' nel '700". In *Sulle tracce della taranta. Documenti inediti del Settecento*. Bari: Regione Puglia, 2000.

Charcot, Jean Martin. *Leçons du mardi a la Salpêtrière, vol. 1: 1887–1888*. Paris: Lecrosnier et Babé & Progrès medical, 1888.

Charcot, Jean Martin. *Leçons du mardi a la Salpêtrière, vol. 2: 1888–1889*. Paris: Lecrosnier et Babé & Progrès medical, 1889.

Charcot, Jean Martin. "Accès d'automatisme ambulatoire de nature comitiale". *Bulletin Médical* 3 (1888): 275–276.

Charcot, Jean Martin. "Ambulatory Automatism". *Medical News* 52 (1888): 309–312.

Chodorow, Nancy J. "Heterosexuality as a Compromise Formation: Reflections on the Psychoanalytic Theory of Sexual Development". *Psychoanalysis and Contemporary Thought* 15/3 (1992): 267–304.

Collins, Randall. "Micro-sociology of Mass Rampage Killings". *Revue de synthèse*, 135/4 (2008): 405–420.

Collins, Randall. *Violence*. Princeton, NJ: Princeton University Press, 2008.

Corraze, Jacques. "La question de l'hystérie". In *A New History of Psychiatry (Nouvelle histoire de la psychiatrie*, edited by Jacques Postel and Claude Quétel, 283–294. Paris: Dunod, 1994.

Costa, Angiola M. *Psicologia sovietica*. Turin: Boringhieri, 1963.

Courtney, J. W. "On the clinical differentiation of the various forms of ambulatory automatism". *The Journal of Abnormal Psychology* 1/3 (1906): 123.

Crepaldi, Marco. *Hikikomori: I giovani che non escono di casa*. Rome: Alpes, 2019.

Czaplinka, Marya Antonina. *Shamanism in Siberia. Excerpts from Aboriginal Siberia*. Kindle edition. Brighton: Evinity Publishing, 2021. [Original work issued 1914]

Dante Alighieri. *The Divine Comedy: Inferno, Purgatorio, Paradiso*, edited by Robin Kirkpatrick. London: Penguin Classics, 2012.

De Caro, Mario. *Realtà*. Turin: Bollati Boringhieri, 2020.

De Heusch, Luc. *Pourquoi l'épouser?* Paris: Gallimard, 1971.

De Martino, Ernesto. *La terra del rimorso*. Milan: Il Saggiatore, 1961.

De Martino, Ernesto. *Sud e magia*. Milan: Feltrinelli, 1959.

Dennis, Philip A. "Grisi Siknis entre los miskitos". *Wani* 24 (1999): 5–12.

Devereux, Georges. "Normal and Abnormal: The Key Problem of Psychiatric Anthropology". In *Some Uses of Anthropology Theoretical and Applied*, edited by Joseph B. Casagrande, and Thomas Gladwin. Washington, DC: Anthropological Society of Washington, 1956.

Di Giuseppe, Mariagrazia, and Perry, John Christopher. "The Hierarchy of Defence Mechanisms: Assessing Defensive Functioning With the Defense Mechanisms Rating Scales Q-Sort". *Frontiers in Psychology* 12 (2021) [https://doi.org/10.3389/fpsyg.2021.718440]

Di Lecce, Giorgio. "Delle tarantole. Dalle cronache medievali alla bibliografia del Settecento". In *Sulle tracce della taranta. Documenti inediti del Settecento*, 83–94. Bari: Regione Puglia, 2000.
Dibattista, Liborio. *J. M. Charcot and the Language of Neurology (J. M. Charcot e la lingua della neurologia)*. Bari: Cacucci, 2003.
Dick, Lyle. "'Pibloktoq' (Arctic Hysteria): A Construction of European-Inuit Relations?". *Arctic Anthropology* 32/2 (1995): 1–42.
Donath, Julius. "Der epileptische Wandertrieb (Poriomanie". *Archiv für Psychiatrie und Nervenkrankheiten* 32/2 (1899): 335–355.
Donath, Julius. "Weitere Beiträge zur Poriomanie". *Archiv für Psychiatrie und Nervenkrankheiten* 42/2 (1907): 752–760.
Dover, Kenneth J. *Greek Homosexuality*. Cambridge, MA: Harvard University Press, 1978.
Eissler Kurt. *Psychologische Aspekte des Briefwechsels zwischen Freud und Jung*. Stuttgart: Frommann-Holzboog: 1982.
Eliade, Mircea. *Shamanism: Archaic Techniques of Ecstasy*. Princeton, NJ: Princeton University Press 1964. [1st edition 1951]
Ellenberger, Henri. *The Discovery of the Unconscious*. New York: Basics Books, 1970.
Ellis, W. Gilmore. "The Amok of the Malays". *Journal of Mental Science* 39/166 (1893): 325–338.
Epifanio, Ferdinando. *Centum historiae seu observationes et casus medici*. Venice: Apud Thomam Ballionum, 1621.
Esterson, Allen. *Seductive Mirage: An Exploration of the Work of Sigmund Freud*. New York: Open Court, 1993.
Fabrega, Horacio Jr., and Silver, Daniel B. "Some Social and Psychological Properties of Zinacanteco Shamans". *Behavioral Science* 15 (1970): 471–486.
Fantini, Bernardino. "Il tarantismo e il ballo di San Vito fra tradizione popolare e medicina colta nell'età moderna". In *RiMorso. La tarantola tra scienza e letteratura*, 63–95. Nardò: Besa, 2001.
Forget Jean. *Exorcisme*. In *Dictionnaire de théologie catholique*, edited by Alfred Vacant, and Eugène Mangenot, vol. 5, 1762–178. Paris: Letouzey et Ané, 1913.
Foschi, Renato, and Innamorati, Marco. *A Critical History of Psychotherapy*. 2 vols. London: Routledge 2022.
Foschi, Renato. Ed. *La libertà sospesa. Il trattamento sanitario obbligatorio e le morti invisibili*. Rome: Fefè 2012.
Foucault, Michel. *History of Madness*. London: Routledge, 2009. [Original work issued 1969]
Frances, Allen. *Saving Normal: An Insider's Revolt Against Out-of-Control Psychiatric Diagnosis*. Boston, MA: Mariner Books, 2013.
Frank, Jerome. *Persuasion and Healing*. Baltimore, MD: Johns Hopkins University Press, 1961.
Freud, Sigmund. "An Autobiographical Study". In *The Standard Edition of the Complete Psychological Works of Sigmund Freud*, edited by James Strachey, vol. 20. London: Hogarth Press. [Original work issued 1924]
Freud, Sigmund. "Civilisation and Its Discontents". In *The Standard Edition of the Complete Psychological Works of Sigmund Freud*, edited by James Strachey, vol. 21. London: Hogarth Press, 1961. [Original work issued 1929]
Freud, Sigmund. "Further Remarks on the Neuro-Psychoses of Defence". In *The Standard Edition of the Complete Psychological Works of Sigmund Freud*, edited by James Strachey, vol. 3. London: Hogarth Press, 1962. [Original work issued 1896].
Freud, Sigmund. "Heredity and the Aetiology of the Neuroses". In *The Standard Edition of the Complete Psychological Works of Sigmund Freud*, edited by

James Strachey, vol. 3. London: Hogarth Press, 1962. [Original work issued 1896]
Freud, Sigmund. "On the History of the Psychoanalytic Movement". In *The Standard Edition of the Complete Psychological Works of Sigmund Freud*, edited by James Strachey, vol. 14. London: Hogarth Press, 1957. [Original work issued 1914]
Freud, Sigmund. "Some General Remarks on Hysterical Attacks". In *The Standard Edition of the Complete Psychological Works of Sigmund Freud*, edited by James Strachey, vol. 9. London: Hogarth Press, 1959. [Original work issued 1908]
Freud, Sigmund. "The Neuro-Psychoses of Defence". In *The Standard Edition of the Complete Psychological Works of Sigmund Freud*, edited by James Strachey, vol. 3. London: Hogarth Press, 1962. [Original work issued 1894]
Freud, Sigmund. "The Psychopathology of Everyday Life". In *The Standard Edition of the Complete Psychological Works of Sigmund Freud*, edited by James Strachey, vol. 6. London: Hogarth Press, 1960. [Original work issued 1901]
Freud, Sigmund. "The Question of a *Weltanschauung*". In *The Standard Edition of the Complete Psychological Works of Sigmund Freud*, edited by James Strachey, vol. 22. London: Hogarth Press, 1964. [Original work issued 1932]
Freud, Sigmund. *Zur Auffassung der Aphasien. Eine Kritische Studie*. Leipzig-Wien: Deuticke, 1891.
Fromm, Erich. *The Fear of Freedom*. London: Routledge, 1941.
Gabbard, Glenn O., and Lester, Eva P. *Boundaries and Boundary: Violations in Psychoanalysis*. New York: Basic Books, 1995.
Gabbard, Glenn O. *Psychodynamic Psychiatry in Clinical Practice*. Washington, DC-London: American Psychiatry Press, 1990.
Gadamer, Hans Georg. *Wahrheit und Methode*. Tübingen: Mohr Siebeck, 1960.
Galimberti, Umberto. "Introduction" to Ernesto De Martino. *La terra del rimorso*. Milan: Il Saggiatore, 2000.
Gallini, Clara. *I rituali dell'àrgia*. Padua: CEDAM, 1967.
Gannushkin, Pyotr B. *Clinical Aspects of Psychopathies, Symptomatics, Dynamics, Systematization*. Moscow: Medgiz, 1933.
Gimlette, John D. "Notes on a Case of Amok". *Journal of Tropical Medicine* 15 (1901): 195–199.
Glover, Edward. *Psycho-analysis. A Handbook for Medical Practitioners and Students of Comparative Psychology*. London-New York: Staples Press, 1949.
Glover, Edward. *The Roots of Crime*. New York: International Universities Press, 1960.
Goetz, Cristopher G. "Charcot at the Salpêtrière: Ambulatory Automatisms". *Neurology*, 37/6 (1987): 1084–1084.
Goetz, Cristopher G., and Klawans, Harold L. "Gilles de la Tourette on Tourette Syndrome". In *Gilles de la Tourette Syndrome*, edited by Arnold J. Friedhoff, and Thomas N. Chase, 1–16, New York: Raven Press, 1982.
Goetz, Cristopher G., and Klawans, Harold L. "Gilles de la Tourette on Tourette Syndrome". *Advances in Neurology* 35 (1982), 1–16.
Goldstein, Jan E. *Console and Classify*. Chicago: University of Chicago Press, 1989.
Goodall, J. *The Chimpanzees of Gombe: Patterns of Behaviour*. Cambridge, MA: Harvard University Press, 1986.
Griesinger, Wilhelm, *Mental Pathology and Therapy*. London: The New Sydenham Society, 1867.
Groddeck, Georg. *The Book of the Id*. New York: Vintage Books, 1949. [Original work issued 1923]
Hacking, Ian. *Façonner les gens (II)*. Course held at the Collège de France in the academic year 2004–2005. [freely accessible at https://www.college-de-france.fr/fr/agenda/cours/faconner-les-gens-ii]

Hacking, Ian. *Mad Travellers: Reflections on the Reality of Transient Mental Illnesses*. Cambridge, MA: Harvard University Press, 1998.
Hacking, Ian. *Rewriting the Soul. Multiple Personality and the Sciences of Memory*. Princeton, NJ: Princeton University Press, 1995.
Halperin, David M. *One Hundred Years of Homosexuality and Other Essays on Greek Love*. London: Routledge, 1990.
Hanson, Norwood Russell. *Patterns of Discovery: An Inquiry into the Conceptual Foundations of Science*. Cambridge: Cambridge University Press, 1959.
Hatta, S. Mohamed. "A Malay Cross-cultural Worldview and Forensic Review of Amok". *Australian & New Zealand Journal of Psychiatry* 30/4 (1996): 505–510.
Heidegger, Martin. *Sein und Zeit*. In *Gesamtausgabe*, vol. 2. Frankfurt am Main: Verlag Vittorio Klostermann, 2024. [Original work issued 1927]
Heinze, Ulrich, and Thomas, Penelope. "Self and Salvation: Visions of Hikikomori in Japanese Manga. *Contemporary Japan* 26/1 (2014): 151–169.
Henshall, Kenneth G. *Japanese Society: Gender, Margins and Mainstream*. New York: St. Martins, 1999.
Herzog, Dagmar. *Cold War Freud*. Cambridge: Cambridge University Press, 2016.
Higgs, Rachel D. "Pibloktoq: A Study of a Culture-bound Syndrome in the Circumpolar Region". *The Macalester Review* 1/1 (2011): 1–9.
Hiyama, Toru, and Yoshihara, Masaharu. "New Occupational Threats to Japanese Physicians: Karoshi (Death due to Overwork) and Karojisatsu (Suicide due to Overwork)". *Occupational and Environmental Medicine* 65/6 (2008): 428–429.
Hobsbawm, Eric J. *The Age of Extremes: The Short Twentieth Idea, 1914–1991*. London: Penguin Michael Joseph, 1994.
Hodges, Andrew. *Alan Turing: The Enigma*. Princeton, NJ: Princeton University Press, 1983.
Hodgkinson, Sarah, H. Prins, and J. Stuart-Bennett. "Monsters, Madmen… and Myths: A Critical Review of the Serial Killing Literature". *Aggression and Violent Behaviour* 34 (2017): 282–289.
Hofstadter, Douglas. *Gödel, Escher, Bach: An Eternal Golden Braid*. New York: Basic Books, 1979.
Husserl, Edmund. "Ideas Pertaining to a Pure Phenomenology and to a Phenomenological Philosophy". In *Collected Works*, vol. 2 (translator F. Kersten). Leiden: Martinus Nijhoff Publishers [Original work published 1913]
Imai, Hissei, Yasuke Ogawa, Kiyohito Okumiya, and Kozo Matsubayashi. "Amok. A Mirror of Time and People: A Historical Review of literature". *History of Psychiatry* 30/1 (2019): 38–57.
Innamorati, Marco, and Rossi, Alessandro. *La rete dell'odio*. Rome: Walter Casini, 2004.
Innamorati, Marco. *Freud*. Rome: Carocci, 2015.
Innamorati, Marco. *Jung*. Rome: Carocci, 2013.
Janet, Pierre, "Les actes inconscients et le dédoublement de la personnalité pendant le somnambulisme provoqué". *Revue Philosophique de la France et de l'Étranger* 22 (1886): 577–592.
Janet, Pierre. *L'automatisme psychologique*. 2 vols. London: Routledge, 2022. [Original work issued 1889]
Jaspers, Karl. *General Psychopathology*, edited by J. Koenig, and Marianne Hamilton. Manchester: Manchester University Press, 1963. [Original work issued 1913]
Jochelson, Waldemar. *Material Culture and Social Organisation of the Koryak: 1905–1908*. New York: Brill, 1908.
Jung, Carl Gustav. "Psychological Types". In *The Collected Works of C. G. Jung*, edited by Herbert Read, Michael Fordham, and Gerhard Adler, vol. 6, 3–495. London: Routledge and Keagan Paul, 1971. [Original work issued issued 1921]

Jung, Carl Gustav. "On the Psychology and Pathology of So-called Occult Phenomena". In *The Collected Works of C. G. Jung*, edited by Herbert Read, Michael Fordham, and Gerhard Adler, vol. 1, 3–88. London: Routledge and Keagan Paul, 1957. [Original work issued issued 1902]

Jung, Carl Gustav. "The Psychology of Dementia Praecox". In *The Collected Works of C. G. Jung*, edited by Herbert Read, Michael Fordham, and Gerhard Adler, vol. 3, London: Routledge and Keagan Paul, 1960. [Original work issued 1907]

Kato, Takahiro A., Ryota Hashimoto, Kohei Hayakawa, Hiroaki Kubo, Motoki Watabe, Alan R. Teo, and Sighenobu Kamba. "Multidimensional Anatomy of 'Modern Type Depression' in Japan: A Proposal for a Different Diagnostic Approach to Depression beyond the DSM-5". *Psychiatry and Clinical Neurosciences* 70 (2016): 7–23.

Kato, Takahiro A., Naotaka Shinfuku, Norman Sartorius, and Shigenobu Kanba. "Loneliness and Single-person Households: Issues of Kodokushi and Hikikomori in Japan". In *Mental Health and Illness in the City*, edited by Niels Okkels, Christina Blanner Kristiansen, and Povl Munk-Jørgensen, 205–219. Singapore: Springer Singapore, 2017.

Kato, Takahiro. A., Naotaka Shinfuku, Norman Sartorius, and Shigenobu Kanba. "Are Japan's Hikikomori and Depression in Young People Spreading Abroad?" *The Lancet* 378/9796 2011): 1070.

Kelly, Henry A. *Towards the Death of Satan: The Growth and Decline of Christian Demonology*. London: Geoffrey Chapman, 1968.

Kenny, Michael G. "Paradox Revisited: Recent Work on the Latah Problem". *Transcultural Psychiatric Research Review* 33/1 (1996): 43–54.

Kerbikov, Oleg V. *The Selected Papers*. Moscow: Meditsina, 1971.

Kernberg, Otto F. *Severe Personality Disorders*. London-New Haven: Yale University Press, 1984.

Kernberg, Otto F., and Caligor, Eve. "A Psychoanalytic Theory of Personality Disorders". In *Major Theories of Personality Disorders*, edited by Mark F. Lenzenweger, and John F. Clarkin, 114–156. New York: Guilford Press, 2005.

Kinsey, Alfred C., Wardell B. Pomeroy, Clyde E. Martin, and Paul H. Gebhard. *Sexual Behaviour in the Human Female*. Philadelphia, PA: W. B. Saunders, 1953.

Kinsey, Alfred C. Wardell B. Pomeroy, and Clyde E. Martin. *Sexual Behaviour in the Human Male*. Philadelphia, PA: W. B. Saunders, 1948.

Kolakowski, Leszek. "Il diavolo". In *Enciclopedia Einaudi*, vol. 4, 703–725. Turin: Einaudi, 1978.

Koryagin, Anatoly. "Unwilling Patients". *The Lancet* 317/8224 (1981): 821–824.

Koyama, Asuka, Yuko Miyake, Norito Kawakami, Masao Tsuchiya, Hisateru Tachimori, Tadashi Takeshima, and World Mental Health Japan Survey Group. "Lifetime Prevalence, Psychiatric Comorbidity and Demographic Correlates of 'Hikikomori' in a Community Population in Japan". *Psychiatry Research* 176/1 (2010): 69–74.

Kraepelin, Emil. "Psychiatrisches aus Java". *Zentralblatt für Nervenheilkunde und Psychiatrie* 27 (1904): 468–469.

Kraepelin, Emil. *Lehrbuch der psychiatrie*. Leipzig: Barth, 1896. [5th edition]

Kraepelin, Emil. *Lehrbuch der psychiatrie*. Leipzig: Barth, 1899. [6th edition]

Krafft Ebing, Richard Von. *Psychopathia Sexualis mit besonderer Berücksichtigung der konträren Sexualempfindung*. Stuttgart: Enke, 1886.

Kua, Ee Heok. "Amok in Nineteenth-century British Malaya History". *History of Psychiatry* 2/4 (1991): 429–436.

Laing, Ronald D. *The Divided Self*. London: Penguin Books, 1959.

Lando, Ortensio. *Commentario delle più notabili e monstruose cose d'Italia e altri luoghi. Catalogo de gli inventori delle cose che si mangiano & si bevono*. Bologna: Pendragon, 1994. [Original work issued 1548]

Lavretsky, Helen. "The Russian Concept of Schizophrenia: A Review of the Literature". *Schizophrenia Bulletin* 24/4 (1998): 537–557.

Lenzenweger, Mark F., and Clarkin, John F. Eds. *Major Theories of Personality Disorder*. New York: Guilford Press, 2005.

Lévi Strauss, Claude. *Structural Anthropology*, vol. 2, edited by Monique Layton. New York: Basic Books, 1963. [Original work issued 1958]

Levy, Jerrold E., Raymond Neutra, and Dennis Parker. "Life Careers of Navajo Epileptics and Convulsive Hysterics". *Social Science & Medicine. Part B: Medical Anthropology* 13/1 (1979): 53–66.

Lewin, Kurt. *A Dynamic Theory of Personality*. New York: McGraw-Hill, 1935.

Lewis, Ioan M. *Ecstatic Religion: An Anthropological Study of Spirit Possession and Shamanism*. London: Penguin Books, 1971.

Lhermitte, Jean. "Les pseudo-possessions diaboliques". In *Études Carmélitaines, Satan*, 213–224. Paris: Desclée de Brouwer, 1948.

Li, Tim M. H., and Wong, Paul W.C. "Youth Social Withdrawal Behaviour (Hikikomori): A Systematic Review of Qualitative and Quantitative Studies". *Australian & New Zealand Journal of Psychiatry* 49/7 (2015): 595–609.

Liddell, Henry G., and Scott, Robert. *A Greek-English Lexicon*. Oxford: Oxford University Press, 1925.

Lingiardi, Vittorio, and Madeddu, Fabio. *I meccanismi di difesa*. Milan: Raffaello Cortina, 2002.

Lingiardi, Vittorio, and McWilliams, Nancy. Eds. *Psychodynamic Diagnostic Manual PDM-2*. New York: Guilford Press, 2017.

Lingiardi, Vittorio. *Citizen Gay*. Milan: Il Saggiatore, 2016.

Loewenstein, Richard J. "Psychogenic Amnesia and Fugue: A Comprehensive Review". *Review of Psychiatry* 10 (1849): 189–222.

Logan, James Richardson. "Malay Amoks and Piracies". *Journal of the Indian Archipelago and Eastern Asia* 3 (1849): 463–467.

Luther, David A., and Derryberry, Elizabeth P. "Birdsongs Keep Pace with City Life: Changes in Song Over Time in an Urban Songbird Affects Communication". *Animal Behaviour* 83/4 (2012): 1059–1066.

Macmillan, Malcolm. *Freud Evaluated: The Completed Arc*. Amsterdam: Elsevier, 1991.

Malagón-Amor, Ángeles, David Córcoles-Martínez, Luis M. Martín-López, and Victor Pérez-Solà. "Hikikomori in Spain: A Descriptive Study". *International Journal of Social Psychiatry* 61/5 (2015): 475–483.

Manzoli, Antonio Maria. "La più antica relazione sulla tarantola. Una lettera del modenese A. M. Manzoli, vescovo di Gravina, a Ulisse Aldrovandi". In *Morso, morbo, morte. La tarantola fra cultura medica e terapia popolare*, edited by Angelo Turchini, 201–203. Milan: Franco Angeli, 1987. [Original work issued 1590]

Marquart, Xavier F. "L'exorciste dans les manifestations diaboliques". In *Études Carmélitaines, Satan*, 328–351. Paris: Desclée de Brouwer, 1948.

Marx, Karl. *Economic and Philosophic Manuscripts of 1844*. New York: International Publishers, 1964.

Mattioli, Pietro Andrea. *I discorsi nelli sei libri di Pedacio Dioscoride Anarzabeo della materia medicinale*. Rome: Julia, 1967. [Original work issued 1548]

McLynn, Frank. *Carl Gustav Jung*. London: Bantam, 1996.

Mecacci, Luciano. *Il caso Marylin M. e altri disastri della psicoanalisi* [*The Marylin M. Case and Other Disasters of Psychoanalysis*]. Rome-Bari: Laterza, 2002.

Melekhov, Dmitri E., S. A. Shubina, and S. E. Kogan. Eds. *Schizophreniya s intericheskimy proyaveniyamy. Troody Inta im.* vol. 1. Moscow: Gannuschkina, 1936.

Midelfort, H. C. Erik. *Exorcism and Enlightenment: Johann Joseph Gassner and the Demons of Eighteenth-century Germany*. New Haven, CT: Yale University Press, 2005.

Miller, David. *A Theory of Shopping*. Cambridge: Polity Press, 1998.
Montanari, Walter. "Il cibo dello sciamano. Etiologia alimentare di una (possibile) sindrome culturale: l'isteria artica". *Cibo e cultura*, edited by Giovanna Motta, vol. 1, 267–280. Rome: Edizioni Nuova Cultura, 2017.
Montinaro, Brizio. *Salento povero*. Ravenna: Longo, 1976.
Montini, Giovanni Battista [Pope Paul VI]. *Insegnamenti*. Rome: Libreria Editrice Vaticana, 1972.
Nietzsche, Friedrich. *Also sprach Zarathustra: Ein Buch für Alle und Keinen*. Chemnitz: Ernst Schmeitzner, 1882–1884.
Nijenhuis, Ellert R. S. *Somatoform Dissociation: Phenomena, Measurement, & Theoretical Issues*. New York: W.W. Norton & Company, 2004.
Nussbaum, Martha. "Preface" to Craig A. Williams. *Roman Homosexuality*, ix–xiv. Oxford: Oxford University Press, 2010.
Onians, Richard B. *The Origins of European Thought*. Cambridge: Cambridge University Press, 1954.
Othmer, Ekkehard, Othmer, Sieglinde. *The Clinical Interview Using DSM-IV-TR: Vol. 1. Fundamentals*. Arlington, VA: APA, 2002.
Palmisano, Antonio Luigi. "Presenza, assenza e rappresentazione nelle trance rituali". In *The Tarantula Between Science and Literature (RiMorso. La tarantola tra scienza e letteratura)*, 137–151. Nardò: Besa, 2001.
Payne, T. R. *S. L. Rubinstein and the Philosophical Foundations of Soviet Psychology*. Dordrecht-New York: Humanities Press, 1968.
Pepe, Roberto, Alberto Durante, and Stefania Panzera. "Il tarantismo: i responsabili". In *Sulle tracce della taranta. Documenti inediti del Settecento*, 113–118. Bari: Regione Puglia, 2000.
Perry, John Christopher. *Defense Mechanism Rating Scales (DMRS)*. Cambridge, MA: J. C. Perry, 1990. [5th edition]
Peters Edward N., Ed. *The 1917 or Pio-Benedictine Code of Canon Law: In English Translation with Extensive Scholarly Apparatus*. San Francisco, CA: Ignatius Press, 2001.
Philippeau, Henri René. *Exorcisme*. In *Catholicism: Yesterday, Today, Tomorrow* [*Catholicisme. Hier, Aujourd'hui, Demain*], edited by Gabriel Jacquemet, vol. 4, 941–945. Paris: Letouzay et Ané, 1956.
Pichot, Pierre. *A Century of Psychiatry* [*Un siècle de psychiatrie*]. Paris: Synthélabo, 1996.
Pick, Daniel. *Faces of Degeneration*. Cambridge: Cambridge University Press, 1989.
Pietikäinen, Petteri. *Madness. A History*. London: Routledge, 2015.
Plas, Régine. *Naissance d'une science humaine, la psychologie: les psychologues et le "merveilleux psychique"*. Rennes: PU Rennes, 2000.
Plato. *Symposium*. In *Lysis – Symposium – Gorgias*, edited by W. R. M Lamb, 73–245. Cambridge, Mass. - London: Harvard University Press, 1925.
Plato. *The Apology of Socrates. A Revised Text and English Notes*, edited by James Riddell. New York: Arno Press, 1973.
Plutarch. *Life of Pelopidas*. In: *The Lives of the Noble Grecians and Romans*, translated by John Dryden, J., edited by Arthur Hugh Clough, 347–367. New York: The Modern Library, 1932.
Plutarch. *The Dialogue on Love*. In *Moralia*, edited by Edwin L. Minar jr., F. H. Sandbach, and W. C. Helmbond, vol. 9, 303–441. Cambridge, Mass. and London: Harvard University Press, 1961.
Popper, Karl Raimund. *The Logic of Scientific Discovery*. London: Routledge, 1959.
Porter, Roy. *Madness. A Brief History*. Oxford-New York: Oxford University Press, 2002.
Postel, Jacques, and Quétel, Claude. Eds. *A New History of Psychiatry* [*Nouvelle histoire de la psychiatrie*]. Paris: Dunod, 1994.

Putnam, Frank W. *Dissociation in Children and Adolescents*. New York: Guilford Press, 1997.
Raffles, Thomas Stamford. *The History of Java*. vol. 1. Oxford: Oxford University Press and Kuala Lumpur, 1828.
Rank, Otto. *The Double. A Psychoanalytic Study* [*Der Doppelgänger*]. London: Karnac Books, 1989. [Original work issued 1914]
Régis, Etienne. "Dromomanie des dégénérés". *Annales Médico-Psychologiques* 8/2 (1895): 204–213.
Rhoades, George. F. jr. "Cross-cultural Aspects of Trauma and Dissociation". *Journal of Trauma Practice* 4 (2005): 21–33.
Ricci, Carla. Ed. *Hikikomori. Narrazioni da una porta chiusa*. Rome: Aracne, 2009.
Ricci, Carla, and Piotti, Antonio. *Hikikomori: adolescenti in volontaria reclusione*. Milan: Franco Angeli, 2008.
Ripa, Cesare. *Iconologia*. Turin: Einaudi, 2012. [Original work issued 1603]
Rituale Romanum: Editio Princeps. Città del Vaticano: Libreria Editrice Vaticana 2004. [Original work issued 1614]
Rossi, Annabella. *Letters from a Tarantata* [*Lettere da una tarantata*]. Bari: De Donato, 1970.
Rothbart, Mary K., Stephan A. Ahadi, and David E. Evans. "Temperament and Personality: Origins and Outcomes". *Journal of Personality and Social Psychology* 78/1 (2000): 122–135.
Rouget, Gilbert. *Music and Trance*. Chicago, IL: The Chicago University Press, 1980.
Rudder Baker, Lynne. *Naturalism and the First-Person Perspective*. Oxford-New York: Oxford University Press, 2013.
Saito, Tamaki. *Hikikomori: Adolescence Without End*. Minneapolis, MN-London: University of Minnesota Press, 2013. [Original work issued 1998]
Saito, Tamaki. "Preface" to *Hikikomori: Adolescence Without End*, 3–8. Minneapolis, MN-London: University of Minnesota Press, 2013.
Sappho, *Lyrics in the Original Greek with Translations*, edited by Willis Barnstone. Garden City NY: Doubleday, 1965.
Savelli, Matt, and Marks, Sarah. Eds. *Psychiatry in Communist Europe*. Basingstoke: MacMillan, 2016.
Scharfetter, Christian. *General Psychopathology*. Cambridge: Cambridge University Press, 2002. [Original work issued 1980]
Schmid, David. *Natural Born Celebrities: Serial Killers in American Culture*. Chicago, IL: University of Chicago Press, 2005.
Schmidt, Karl, Lee Hill, and George Guthrie. "Running Amok". *International Journal of Social Psychiatry*, 23/4 (1977): 264–274.
Schmidtke, Armin, Sylvia Schaller, and Laura Müller. "Imitation of Amok and Amok-suicide". *Kritz Dergisi*, 10 (2002): 49–60.
Scull, Andrew. *Madness in Civilisation: A Cultural History of Insanity From the Bible to Freud, From the Madhouse to Modern Medicine*. Princeton, NJ: Princeton University Press, 2015.
Serao, Francesco, *Della Tarantola o sia Falangio di Puglia*. Nardò: Salento Books, 2007. [Original work published 1742].
Shamdansani, Sonu. *Jung Stripped Bare by His Biographers, Even*. London: Karnac Books, 2005.
Sieroszevski, Waclav. "Du chamanisme d'après les croyances des Yakoutes". *Revue de l'histoire des religions*, 46 (1902): 204–235; 299–338.
Sigerist, Henry E. "The Story of Tarantism". In *Medicine and Music*, edited by Dorothy M. Schullian, and Max Schoen, 96–116. New York: Schuman, 1948.
Simon, Linda. *Genuine Reality: A Life of William James*. New York-San Diego-London: Harcourt Brace and Company, 1998.

Smith, Theresa C., and Oleszczuk, Thomas. A. *No Asylum*. London: Palgrave Macmillan, 1996.
Smulevich, A. B. "Sluggish Schizophrenia in the Modern Classification of Mental Illness". *Schizophrenia Bulletin* 15/4 (1989): 533–539.
Solito, Domenico. *Descrizione storico-filosofica delle più rinomate conchiglie che allignano nel seno tarantino e della famigerata tarantola di Puglia: con un Cenno storico sulla fondazione, sul progresso, e decadimento dell'antichissima città di Taranto*. Rome: Zampi, 1845.
Spedicato, Mario. *Chiesa e trasgressione. Tarantismo in terra d'Otranto in età post-tridentina*. In *RiMorso. La tarantola tra scienza e letteratura*, 9–21. Nardò: Besa, 2001.
Spores, John C. *Running Amok*. Athens, OH: Ohio University Center for International Studies and Center for Southeast Asian Studies, 1988.
Sroufe, L. Alan, Brianna Coffino, and Elizabeth A. Carlson. "Conceptualizing the Role of Early Experience: Lessons from the Minnesota Longitudinal Study". *Developmental Review* 30/1 (2010): 36–51.
Staff, Jeremy. "Coming of Age in America: The Transition to Adulthood in the Twenty-first Century". *Contemporary Sociology: A Journal of Reviews* 42 (2013): 117–118.
Stern, Paul J. *C. G. Jung: The Haunted Prophet*. New York: George Braziller, 1978.
Stevenson, Robert Louis. *The Strange Case of Dr Jekyll and Mr Hyde*. London: Longmans, Green and Co, 1886.
Stoller, Robert J. *Sex and Gender*. London: Karnac Books, 1984. [Original work issued 1968]
Straus, Erwin. *Phenomenological Psychology*. New York: Grune & Stratton, 1968.
Strenger, Carlo. *Between Hermeneutics and Science: Psychological Issues*. Madison, CT: International Universities Press, 1991.
Suchareva, Grunya Y. "On the Problems of Defect in the Soft Forms of Schizophrenia". *Soviet Neurology, Psychiatry and Psychohygiene*, 2 (1933): 24–38.
Suryani, Luh Ketut, and Jensen, Gordon D. *Trance and Possession in Bali: A Window on Western Multiple Personality, Possession Disorder, and Suicide*. Oxford: Oxford University Press, 1995.
Suwa, Mami, and Suzuki, Kazuhiro. "The Phenomenon of 'Hikikomori' (Social Withdrawal) and the Socio-cultural Situation in Japan Today". *Journal of Psychopathology* 19 (2013): 191–198.
Swettenham, Frank A. *Malay Sketches*. London: John Lane, 1895.
Swettenham, Frank A. *The Real Malay*. London: Ballantyne, Hanson & Co, 1899.
Sydenham, Thomas "Epistolary Dissertation to Dr. Cole. Presentation copy in the College of Physicians dated March 21, 1682". *European Neurology* 76/3–4 (2016): 175–181.
Taradel, Ruggero *L'accusa del sangue*. Rome: Editori Riuniti, 2002.
Teo, Alan R., Michael D. Fetters, Kyle Stufflebam, Masaru Tateno, Yatan Balhara, Tae Young Choi, Shigenobu Kanba, Carol A. Mathews, and Takahiro A. Kato. "Identification of the Hikikomori Syndrome of Social Withdrawal: Psychosocial Features and Treatment Preferences in Four Countries". *International Journal of Social Psychiatry* 61/1 (2015): 64–72.
Teoh, Jin Inn. "The Changing Psychopathology of Amok". *Psychiatry* 35/4 (1972): 345–351.
Thomas Aquinas, *Summa Theologiae*. In *Aquinas Institute Opera Omnia Project*, edited by The Aquinas Institute and translated by Thomas Shapcote, vols. 13–22. Rochester, NY: Aquinas Institute and Emmaus Academic, 2023.
Throop, C. Jason, and Dornan, Jennifer L. "Psychopathology and Shamanism". In *Shamanism. An Encyclopaedia of World Beliefs, Practices and Culture*, edited by

Mariko Namba Walter and Eva Jane Neumann Fridmann, 211–217. Santa Barbara, CA – Denver, CO – Oxford: ABC-CLIO, 2004.
Thyraeus, Petrus. *Loca Infesta, Hoc est: De Infestis, Ob Molestantes Daemoniorum et Defunctorum Hominvm Spiritus, Locis, Liber Unus ... accessit eiusdem Libellus de Terriculamentis nocturnis, quae hominium mortem solent protendere.* Cologne: Cholinus, 1598.
Timpanaro, Sebastiano. *Il lapsus freudiano. Psicoanalisi e critica testuale.* Florence: La Nuova Italia, 1974.
Tinbergen, Nico. *The Study of Instinct.* Oxford and New York: Oxford University Press, 1952.
Tissié, Philippe Auguste. *Les Aliénés Voyageurs: Le Cas d'Albert.* Paris: L'Harmattan, 2005. [Original work issued 1887]
Tolstoy, Leo. *Anna Karenina.* Oxford: Oxford University Press, 2014. [Original work issued 1877]
Tonquedec, Joseph de. "Quelques aspectes de l'action de Satan dans le monde". In *Études Carmélitaines, Satan*, 493–506. Paris: Desclée de Brouwer, 1948.
Tonquedec, Joseph de. *Les maladies nerveuses ou mentales et les manifestations diaboliques.* Paris, France: Beauchesne, 1938.
Turchini, Angelo. Ed. *Morso, morbo, morte. La tarantola fra cultura medica e terapia popolare.* Milan: Franco Angeli, 1987.
Van Loon, F. H. G. "Amok and Lattah". *The Journal of Abnormal and Social Psychology* 21/4 (1927): 434–444.
Van Voren, Robert. "Political Abuse of Psychiatry: An Historical Overview". *Schizophrenia Bulletin* 36/1 (2010): 33–35.
Van Voren, Robert. Ed. *Soviet Psychiatric Abuse in the Gorbachev Era.* Amsterdam: IAPUP, 1989.
Wallace, Anthony F. C., and Ackerman, Robert E. "An Interdisciplinary Approach to Mental Disorder among the Polar Eskimos of Northwest Greenland". *Anthropologica* 2 (1960): 249–260.
Watanabe, Takeshi. "Il mio mestiere di counseling e hikikomori". In *Hikikomori. Narrazioni da una porta chiusa*, edited by Carla Ricci, 121–134. Rome: Aracne, 2009.
Wehr, Gerhard. *Jung: A Biography.* Boston: Shambala, 1985.
Westen, Drew, Jonathan Shedler, and Vittorio Lingiardi. *La valutazione della personalità con la swap-200.* Milan: Raffaello Cortina, 2014.
Westermeyer, Joseph. "On the Epidemicity of Amok Violence". *Archives of General Psychiatry* 28/6 (1973): 873–876.
Wilde, Oscar, *De Profundis.* New York-London: Putnam, 1905.
Williams, Craig A. *Roman Homosexuality.* Oxford: Oxford University Press, 2010.
Winzeler Robert. *Emotions of Culture.* Singapore-New York: Oxford University Press, 1990.
Winzeler, Robert. *Latah in Southeast Asia: The Ethnography and History of a Culture-bound Syndrome.* Cambridge: Cambridge University Press, 1995.
Wittgenstein, Ludwig. *On Certainty.* Oxford: Basil Blackwell, 1969.
Wittkower, Eric D., and Prince, Raymond. "A Review of Transcultural Psychiatry". In *American Handbook of Psychiatry*, 2 (1974): 335–350.
Wojtila, Karol [Pope John Paul II]. *General Audience. Wednesday, 13 August 1986* [*Udienza Generale. 13 agosto 1986*]. https://w2.vatican.va/content/john-paul-ii/it/audiences/1986/documents/hf_jp-ii_aud_19860813.html.
Wong, Paul W.C. "Social Withdrawal as Invisible Youth Disengagement". *International Journal of Sociology and Social Policy* 32 (2012): 415–430.
World Health Organisation (WHO). *The ICD-10 Classification of Mental and Behavioural Disorders: Diagnostic Criteria for Research.* New York: World Health Organisation, 1993.

Zajicek, Benjamin. "Soviet Madness: Nervousness, Mild Schizophrenia, and the Professional Jurisdiction of Psychiatry in the USSR, 1918-1936". *Ab Imperio* 4 (2014): 167–194.
Zajicek, Benjamin. "Soviet Psychiatry and the Origins of the Sluggish Schizophrenia Concept, 1912–1936". *History of the Human Sciences* 31/2 (2018): 88–105.
Zaner, Richard M. *The Problem of Embodiment: Some Contributions to a Phenomenology of the Body*. The Hague: Springer, 1964.
Zielenziger, Michael. *Shutting Out the Sun: How Japan Created Its Own Lost Generation*. New York: Random House, 2006.
Zweig, Stefan. *Amok*. London: Pushkin Press, 2006. [1st edition 1922]

Index

Note: Gods, characters from the Bible, mythology and works of fiction are shown in italics. The latter and aliases of clinical cases are indicated by their first name before the surname or initial (e.g. Dorian Gray, Félida X). Numbers in italics refer to notes.

FSC
www.fsc.org
MIX
Papier | Fördert gute Waldnutzung
FSC® C083411

Kolibri 360 GmbH
Ferdinand-Jühlke-Straße 7
99095 Erfurt, Deutschland
produktsicherheit@kolibri360.de